# Living with Your Bad Back

## By THEODORE BERLAND

*The Scientific Life*

*Your Children's Teeth*
(WITH ALFRED E. SEYLER, D.D.S.)

*X-ray—Vanguard of Modern Medicine*

*How to Keep Your Teeth After 30*

*The Fight for Quiet*

*Living with Your Ulcer*
(WITH MITCHELL A. SPELLBERG, M.D.)

*Living with Your Bad Back*
(WITH ROBERT G. ADDISON, M.D.)

# LIVING WITH YOUR BAD BACK

## Theodore Berland

### and

## Robert George Addison, M.D., F.A.A.O.S., F.A.C.S., F.I.C.S.

Assistant Professor of Orthopedics,
Northwestern University Medical School
Senior Attending Orthopedic Surgeon,
Chicago Wesley Memorial Hospital
Chairman, Section of Orthopedics,
St. Joseph Hospital, Chicago
Chief, Division of Surgery, Rehabilitation
Institute of Chicago
Medical Consultant, Sealy, Inc.

Illustrations by June Hill Pedigo

ST. MARTIN'S PRESS, INC.
New York City

ST. MARTIN'S PRESS    NEW YORK

© Copyright 1972 by Theodore Berland
All rights reserved.

First Printing

Library of Congress No. 72-166171
Manufactured in the United States of America.
No part of this book may be reproduced without
permission in writing from the publisher.

St. Martin's Press
175 Fifth Avenue
New York, N.Y. 10010

AFFILIATED PUBLISHERS: Macmillan & Company, Limited, London
—also at Bombay, Calcutta, Madras and Melbourne—
the Macmillan Company of Canada, Limited, Toronto

*To my brother, Larry, who inherited
a better back than I.*

T.B.


*For my back patients, so they can
enjoy the fullest measure of life.*

R.G.A.

# Acknowledgments

We wish to thank the American Medical Association Library for providing excellent reference material, and Edith Lovinger, who skillfully and patiently typed the manuscript.

R.G.A.

# Contents

# 1. Ted's Bad Back

As well as he can remember, it all started when Ted was 28. He was teeing off on the fourth hole. The weather was miserable on this public course. He and his friends realized they were rushing the golf season, since it was April, but they were eager to unlimber and start playing again after a confining, snow-filled winter. This early spring Saturday morning the sun was hardly penetrating the ground mist; there was a damp chill in the air.

It was Ted's turn at the tee. He grasped the handle of his driving wood, adjusted his stance, concentrated his attention on the little pock-marked white ball momentarily at rest on the yellow sprout of wood before him on the grass. Carefully he drew back his club, hesitated at the top of the swing and pulled through. As he finished the swing he cried out in pain. His back had suddenly "snapped." He felt a sharp pain in the small of his back. Ted dropped his club, winced and futilely put his hand to his back as if to press out the pain. He explained what had happened to his concerned friends and told

1

them he'd go back to the clubhouse. The walk back, pulling his golf cart, was torturous. Loading his golf clubs in the car, sliding into the seat and driving home provoked special pains.

At home, Ted's wife called a doctor, who told them to meet him at the hospital. There he examined Ted and applied strips of tape to the small of his back. A week or so later, when Ted returned to have the tape removed, the doctor lectured him about having a "trick back" and told him to watch himself, take it easy and try for a game of 100, not 70.

Ted's back behaved for the next three years. Then, on a Christmas weekend, it disabled him again. He and his wife were bowling with some friends. Ted was not a serious bowler, although he had his own ball and shoes. His game that night, as always, was mediocre, but he enjoyed the socializing and conversation and, most of all, watching the women bowl.

After bowling their three lines, the couples left and went to a nearby restaurant for a late snack. Ted found he was uncomfortable at the table; he kept changing positions in his seat. Despite his shuffling, he could not find a position in which his back did not hurt. After some ten minutes of this torture, he turned to his wife and whispered that he really had to go home. They made their apologies and left the restaurant.

Once home, Ted went to bed, mumbling that he was sure he would feel better in the morning. And when he awakened the next day, Sunday, he did feel better. So much better, in fact, that he set about to tidy up the basement. In the late afternoon, his back pain returned rather suddenly when he lifted with his right hand a "portable" 30-pound tape recorder. He set it down again rather quickly. Now his back was not merely uncomfortable. It hurt. Not as it did after the golf mishap—it was a more vague, yet penetrating pain that spread over all the small of his back.

Ted walked upstairs to the kitchen, sat down gingerly, and hoped the pain would go away. It did seem to get better during dinner. Later he took a short walk to a corner delicatessen. It was very cold out, the sidewalks were icy and as he returned home with a bag of Danish sweet rolls, he became aware of a deep pain burning in his back. The pain was very low; in fact, it was almost at his seat.

Home again, he spent the rest of the evening sitting and watching television.

The next morning Ted couldn't roll out of bed. He was awake, but the pain was so sharp that he could not sit up. His wife served him breakfast as he lay flat on his back. Then she called an orthopedic surgeon who was caring for their baby daughter. The doctor suggested they come to his office immediately so that Ted could be examined.

It took all the effort Ted could muster to slink out of bed; get into his clothes with his wife's help; and, to hand-over-hand use her body as support to achieve a posture that approximated standing. With his shoulders slouched, and his back as rigid as a C-clamp, he shuffled one foot in front of the other. With the weight of his hands on the back of his wife's shoulders, he painfully made his way to the car, and then from the car to the doctor's office.

His back continued to hurt as he sat and waited for his turn to see the doctor. And when he was called, he had to again use his wife's body as a support to achieve a standing posture. When the doctor saw Ted, he shook his head in appreciation of the pain. His examination was thorough but rather brief. He noted Ted's too-straight lower back and the rigidity both standing and supine. He explained to Ted that the muscles of his back were in a spasm, which was why he was in pain. The problem was to find the underlying cause of the spasm, perhaps some spinal disorder. To do both—treat the spasm and pain and find the causes—the doctor said Ted should go to the hospital immediately.

With that, the doctor picked up the telephone and called the hospital to arrange for a bed. On their way to the hospital, Ted told his wife he was shocked. And he was confused and frustrated. How would his wife, four months pregnant with their second child, manage without him? And what about his work? He had been on his own for less than three years and unless he worked every day, his income would fall drastically. She assured him that she wasn't surprised, that when he awakened that morning she knew she would have to take him to the hospital. Call it intuition or insight, she was right.

At the hospital, Ted was admitted to a room, undressed and put to bed with a quick hypodermic in his rump to ease his intense pain and calm his fears and tensions.

During his next ten days in the hospital, he was on his back all the time. On the first day he was placed in traction: a cloth device akin to a garter belt was buckled around his waist; attached to its straps was a 15-pound weight at the foot of the bed. Every afternoon he was lifted from his bed, placed on a cart and wheeled to the physical therapy department, where he spent a wonderful, relaxing half-hour with penetrating heat to relax the muscles at the small of his back.

Every morning his doctor, accompanied by a pair of residents, came to see him. They would examine him by raising first one leg, then the other, to measure the pain in the small of Ted's back. After ten days, the doctor said Ted could go home. On the day of his discharge, Ted felt weak and shaky as he sat up in bed unaided and dangled his legs over the side. Then he was taken in a wheel chair to another part of the hospital where the doctor fashioned a plaster cast over his entire trunk, from hips to nipples. The doctor said Ted would be wearing it for a month.

At first, Ted felt like a turtle, enclosed as he was in a rigid shell of plaster. Of course he couldn't bend forward, or even sideward. But he said a silent thanks that he did not suffer from claustrophobia, the fear of enclosure. After a few days on his feet and at his desk, he felt rather comfortable in it. He learned to do many of the things he had to do and liked to do. Some of these activities, such as making love to his wife, required some creativity, but still he managed.

He was also fortunate that he was wearing his cast in the winter when his perspiration rate was at a minimum. Even so, after two weeks, he started to itch a bit now and then. He learned to take a deep breath and blow down the front of his body, in the space created between him and the cast. This gave him some ventilation and kept the itching down. Also, whenever he itched he learned to rotate himself a bit in his cast so as to rub that area of skin against the cloth liner. But there were many times when he would reach to scratch his trunk and his fingers would surprisingly bang against the hard plaster.

When the month was up, Ted visited the doctor at the hospital, where the cast was sawed off. Then Ted was sent to a corset house where he was fitted for a corset which he would wear continuously for a month and every once in a while for the rest of his life.

It has been more than a decade since Ted was hospitalized. His back still pains him occasionally, for a few days at a time, and usually when other things are troubling him too. But he has learned that his back is but one of the pains of life which he must bear. Yet he follows his doctor's advice: he is careful about lifting heavy things, careful in his selection of sports activities, and exercises as regularly as he can.

To Ted his back was unique and singular. It struck him down at a time of his life when he was otherwise vigorous and active. To his doctor, Ted was unique as an individual, but rather ordinary as a patient by virtue of his disorder. Ted suffered essentially two attacks of lower back pain—which, in his father's day, was called acute lumbago. Most back patients suffer one or two attacks, although some have chronic back troubles that cause frequent attacks.

Ted's attacks came after golf, bowling and lifting. Other stories doctors hear begin . . .

"I was leaning over the washbowl, rinsing my face when suddenly it felt as though someone kicked me in the back."

"I was opening a window when I suddenly felt this fire in my legs. Now I walk to one side. And my toes are numb."

"I leaned over to pick up a paper clip and I couldn't straighten up again."

Those who suffer from bad back, including Ted, are among a legion of Americans who mumble about their aching backs and refrain from carrying grips or shoveling snow. One writer, Marshall Smith, estimated in his *Life* magazine article in 1965 that 28 million Americans (30 million, said Associated Press in 1970) suffer from bad backs. He claimed that "the bad back has become more fashionable in this country than the bad liver is in France. It has replaced the ulcer as the badge of high-pressure living. It has emerged as a status symbol that sufferers boldly and openly proclaim." Among famous back sufferers have been such show people as Sophie Tucker, Don Ameche, Elizabeth Taylor and Joe E. Lewis; restaurateur Toots Shor; St. Louis Cardinals shortstop Marty Marion; Frank Gifford, N.Y. Giants star halfback; Sen. Barry Goldwater; and the late President John F. Kennedy.

While few people have died of bad backs, almost all back sufferers will say, during the acute phase of their attack, that they wish they could die and end the pain. The numbers of those who suffer are, indeed, in the millions, according to the most reliable statistics available—those of the National Health Survey. In the 1960's it found that about 5 million Americans suffered from unspecified impairments of the lower back. The surveyors defined these impairments as chronic difficulties including stiffness, weakness, pain trouble, spasms and swellings. But the total does not include such specific low back troubles as slipped disk, compressed nerve and sciatica. Another survey (by the Commission on Professional and Hospital Activities) showed that "disk displacement" is the 16th most prevalent reason for admission to hospitals, and lower back "pains and strains" the 36th.

The National Health Survey data pierce through the smog of rumors and legends about bad back much as vapors of vinegar cut through tobacco smoke. For instance, back trouble hits men with just a little more frequency than it does women (28.3 per thousand for men versus 25.8 per thousand for women). Most back problems are of the kind we're talking about, accounting for some 75 percent of *all* back and spine disorders. Among chronic conditions that limit the activities of Americans at home and at work, bad back rates third—after arthritis-rheumatism and heart trouble. Backs bad enough to limit activity are most troublesome for women under 45 years of age and for men 45 to 64 years. The more money people make, the more likely they are to have bad backs—but this is only a slight edge. Some 6.5 percent of all persons living in families with incomes of less than $3,000 a year are limited in their activities because of bad back; while this is true of 9.2 percent of those in families with incomes of more than $15,000. Age and geography, for some reason, are far more relevant. Middle-aged persons who live in the northern and western United States are twice as likely to have bad backs as are southerners. In fact, in the west bad back is the leading impairment of persons under 65 years of age. Finally, people living on farms, in small towns, or in large cities have equal chances of having bad backs.

On any given day in America, 6.5-million men and women are in bed with low-back trouble. Back injuries are the major industrial disabler: 600,000 workers are away from their jobs during each year because they hurt their backs at work. According to one estimate, this costs their employers about a billion dollars annually in sickpay and in wages for replacement personnel.

His bad back made Ted more than a statistic. As a sufferer, he has a malady that is distinctly human. No other animal has the same back troubles which human beings do, although dachshunds have back problems, too—of another breed.

People have suffered from lumbago and other backaches for centuries. But the term "achin' back" dates historically to World War II, when it was a common complaint of United States servicemen. One explanation for the ubiquity of the malady was the heavy backpack and heavy weapons the soldiers carried. But other soldiers in previous wars also hauled heavy loads of equipment, yet did not phrase their complaint so.

You should, in this day and age, wear your bad back with the same pride as did those servicemen of World War II. Consider it the price you must pay for standing erect; call it another bit of currency exacted from your body for being above the lower animals not only in intellect but in altitude.

Our objective in this book is to give you all of the background and facts you need to understand your lower back and why it hurts; how your problem developed and why your doctor treats it as he does. (We will not be dealing with whiplash, coccyx fractures or disorders of other areas of the back.) In addition to telling you the pertinent anatomy and physiology of your lower back, this book will also give you the details of various kinds of treatment for your back—in the hospital bed, in the operating room and at home. It is not our intent to scare you, but to inform you. We feel that the worst thing would be for you to become a "back cripple" and be so fearful of your condition that you drastically reduce or even stop your activities. Your bad back is something you have to learn to live with. We hope that this book can make that possible and less painful.

We assume that the reader of this book is an adult, and so the information that follows is intended to be conveyed from one adult to another. There is no attempt here to frost with sugar or to substitute cute nicknames for real terms, although where there are popular, commonly used terms for parts of the body or injuries, we will also use these to help your understanding.

As you use this book, remember that it is a tool you should use with good judgment. No book can replace the skills and services of your personal physician. His diagnosis and prescribed plan of treatment must in all cases supersede anything said here. If there is any controversy or contradiction between the words printed here and what he advises, take his word against ours.

On the other hand, the information included here should help spare you the need to ask your doctor to give you a short medical education in the origin, diagnosis and treatment of low back pain. It should also inform you of the facts you want or need but are too rushed or too embarrassed to ask of him. We also hope that this book saves your doctor some time and explanation.

In other words, this book is designed to help you live with your achin' back. If it does that, it will have achieved its purpose and its authors' intention.

# 2. Understanding Your Back

Your spine is a string of 26 bones arranged somewhat like a swaying stack of poker chips. The fact that your spine is vertical puts you in a category of the most advanced creatures on earth, those that stand erect and walk on two hind limbs. Sitting on top of your spine—actually balanced there—is your skull, with its magnificent occupant, the human brain. That brain's creativity, speed and ability to work with many numbers and symbols simultaneously and sequentially, plus its incredible storage system, allow man to be master of the earth and the moon. But he could never strut over his land if his backbone were not erect.

We are members of that group of animals with backbones, a group distinguished by its internal skeletons. Called *vertebrates,* the group includes fishes, amphibians, reptiles, birds and mammals. Vertebrates have been on earth 400 million years, but the longest surviving kind are the fishes, which are 200 million years old. Reptiles, the first vertebrates to live out of water, dominated the scene 100 million years ago. Birds were the first animals able to maintain a constant body temperature. Mammals are also warm-blooded but are relative newcomers, having been around for 55 million years. Modern man, our upright, naked kind of mammal, has been on earth about a million years, although prehuman forms existed five to ten million years ago.

As a vertebrate animal, you are distinct from the other animals—insects, lobsters, spiders, worms, jellyfish, sponges —in that you have a proportionately large trunk and two sets of limbs (or the remnant of limbs: those of snakes and whales disappeared with disuse through the eons). Thanks to their strong internal skeletons, vertebrate animals became the biggest creatures on earth.

If you compare the backbone to the keel of a boat, you can perhaps appreciate this marvelous engineering achievement of nature. Think, for instance, of the immense strength necessary in the backbone of the brachiosaurus dinosaur, which once roamed Wyoming and East Africa. That spine had to carry much of the giant's 50 tons and transmit this weight to its four massive legs. In fact, the dead weight of that column of bones (vertebrae) was itself considerable.

The lowest form of vertebrate animal, the fish, has a straight spine to which is attached a powerful set of muscles. This combination gives the fish its propulsion system: what looks to us landlubbers like a small flick of the trunk and tail is actually a powerful push against the water. In land animals like us, though, the trunk is comparatively weak since it is not used for propulsion. Instead, land animals propel themselves with their legs. To give you some idea of the difference in musculature, look at the meat we eat. Filet of sole is trunk muscle; ham is leg muscle.

Because the trunk muscles are weaker in land animals, the vertebrae are thicker and stronger. Also, because the backbone has to help hold the body off the ground it cannot be as straight as that of a fish. Instead, it is arched, its ends anchored to the front and rear legs in much the same kind of construction as that used in suspension bridges like San Francisco's Golden Gate.

In apes, which walk partially erect some of the time, and in man, who walks fully erect all of the time (except when his back aches), the curvature of the spine is further modified with a second curve. This is most pronounced in the human spine; in order for you to stand vertical, the center of gravity of your body has to be centrally located. That means straight above the hips. To achieve this, your spine curves forward just above the hips and throws the chest (located above it) forward and up. This gives it its characteristis S-shape and its springlike ability to keep the body erect when you walk. Incidentally, a newborn baby's spine is C-shaped; it develops the second curve later when it starts to sit; it is further developed as the child becomes a toddler and walks.

Earlier we said that the backbone is like the keel of a boat. This is less true of your spine than it is of a fish's. Another way to look at your spine is as the bar in a barbell—but a vertical one with one mass at the top and another at the bottom.

The skull is balanced at the top end of the spine. But connected just a bit lower are the shoulders, from which hang the arms. And just below the shoulders are the ribs and their contents. So the upper weight of the body, which the spine holds up, contains the head, chest and upper limbs.

The base of the spine is anchored in the pelvic girdle, that firm ring of flattened bone that rides on your hips. The pelvis and your legs make up the other weight attached to the spine. This means that your spine has to bend and twist between these two masses—anchored in the lower one and balancing the upper one.

Quite a task!

Your spine does even more. This very good summation was given in a medical textbook[1]:

[1]Arthur Steindler, *Mechanics of Normal and Pathological Locomotion in Man* (Springfield: Charles C Thomas, 1935), p. 117.

The main function of the spine is that of a sustaining rod which maintains the upright position of the body and carries its weight. Moreover, it is a balancing rod which is firmly planted into the pelvic ring. It serves as a post of anchorage for the powerful musculature of the shoulder girdle and the upper extremity. It is a casing which encloses the most delicate structure of the body, namely the spinal cord, and it is a post upon which the thoracic cage is suspended and upon which it depends very largely for its respiratory function. It is a buffer spring which receives and distributes in rapid and endless sequence innumerable jars and jolts associated with dynamic functions of the body. It is also an organ of great flexibility which produces moments of force and receives, concentrates and transmits those originating in other parts of the body. In order to fulfill these varied functions the construction of the spine must be such as to satisfy the most intricate static as well as dynamic demands.

Being all back, a snake has about 300 vertebrae; you have approximately one-tenth as many. Your spine began to form when you were an embryo a mere three weeks after your conception. Two weeks later your vertebrae began to form as separate bones. When you were born your spine had 33 separate vertebrae and they still hadn't closed, so your spinal cord was exposed. The slit closed in the first few years, while you were an infant. During your years of growing up, the four bones at the bottom end of the spine, your vestigial tail, fused together to form one of the body's few useless bones, called the *coccyx*. The five bones above the tail, those connected to the pelvis, also fused; this second solid portion of the spine is called the *sacrum*.

From here up, the spine moves. The five vertebrae above the sacrum, which form the forward curve at the small of your back are the lumbar vertebrae. (This forward curve is called *lordosis,* after the haughty mien of a lord!) The next 12, which form a curve backwards are the *thoracic,* or

chest, vertebrae to which your ribs are connected. Riding
highest on your spine are the seven cervical vertebrae of your
neck, the topmost of which is the atlas, so-called because,
like the ancient titan, it supports a globe—in this case the
head.

Doctors use a shorthand to refer to each of the vertebrae.
Composed of a letter and a number, it is rather simple to
decipher once you understand it. The letter is an initial for
the segment of the spine: cervical, thoracic, or lumbar. The
numbering starts at the top of each segment. The ones you
probably will hear about most frequently are L4 and L5—

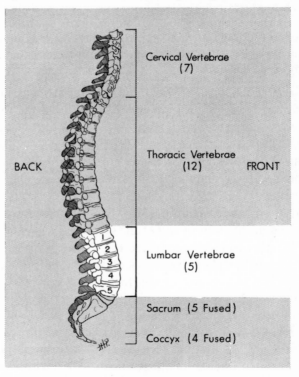

*The human spine. The lumbar vertebrae at the small of the*
*back are the ones that most often cause problems.   Fig. 1*

the fourth and fifth lumbar vertebrae. The connection between L5 and the sacrum is called the lumbosacral joint. It is important to know this because it is a frequent source of backache.

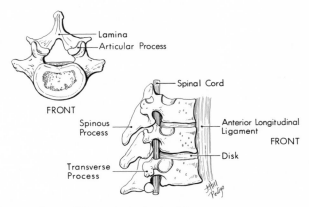

*The vertebrae. These complicated bones rest one on top of the other and have gelatinlike cushions, or disks, between them.* **Fig. 2**

Your 24 moveable vertebrae are complicated bones. The rear half of each is made of several smaller bones fused into a crude **W** shape, which is connected to the front part of the vertebra, a thick circular bone. Looked at in silhouette from the top or bottom, each vertebra could be construed to be a Western brand of the fictional Circle-W Ranch! The vertebrae look different from the side, however, because the "wings" of the **W** *(transverse processes)* are horizontal, while the center of the **W** angles downward. That center projection is called the *spinous process* and is what you feel when you rub your fingertip down the center of your back. Coming from each transverse process are projections *(articular processes),* which stick up and down; these are the parts of the vertebrae that rub against each other and support each other and that can be the site of such troubles as arthritis. Also, the bones that make up the W usually break first when the back suffers a blow or a fall.

The bottom of the W forms a round hole through which passes the most sensitive part of your body: your spinal cord. It is, in effect, your master trunkline of nerves, carrying sensations from various parts of the body to your brain and carrying commands from your brain out to various parts of your body—organs, muscles, glands. Nerves branch off from the spinal cord and pass between vertebrae at appropriate levels—to the neck, arms, chest, abdomen and legs. Nerves also go to the muscles that move the spine, which are connected to the center and wings of the bony W—the spinous and transverse processes. When the trunkline is severed, through an automobile accident or in combat, the result can be loss of feeling and the ability to move. If both legs are paralyzed it is called paraplegia. When the damage is higher, affecting the arms as well, it is called quadraplegia.

The body of each vertebra is kept separate and cushioned from its neighbors above and below by *disks,* which are pads of tough cartilage, or gristle. These form a joint that permits limited motion, such as bending and twisting, but is not as free as such fluid-bathed joints as your knee. Because they are somewhat elastic, the intervertebral disks also act as shock absorbers; that, plus the springlike action of your spine as you walk, helps prevent your brain from having a concussion with every step you take.

These disks account for about one-fourth of the total length of your spine. Because of the squeezing and pounding they get in the course of a day's walking, bending, sitting and twisting, your disks are slightly compressed by the time you go to bed. In fact, you are probably three-fourths of an inch shorter than when you awaken in the morning. Furthermore, it is the disks, or what happens to them, that explain why people seem to get shorter as they get older.

You are tallest when you are at the peak of your growth,

somewhere in the late teens, perhaps 18 years old. As you get older, the disks dry out; it is part of the aging process and occurs without your perceiving it. One factor is the wear they take with every day's and every minute's use. Another is the hormonal changes that come in later life as the body shifts its endocrine gears from build-up to level-off or even to breakdown. This affects not only the disks, but the vertebrae (and other bones) as well. As a result of these effects of aging, your disks narrow as you get older, so that when you retire you will be one to two inches shorter than when you started your career or your housekeeping. Thus when you go to bed as a senior citizen you may be three inches shorter than you were as a youth getting up in the morning. If, as you age, you start stooping and you become roundbacked (widow's hump, it is called in post-menopausal women) you will be even shorter—perhaps another 8 to 10 inches shorter.

Taking a closer look at a healthy disk, its center (or *nucleus pulposus*) has a consistency resembling that of a slightly stale gum drop. Its "skin" is a tough ring of fibers called the *annulus fibrosis*. When the disk becomes diseased and deteriorates, it becomes white and shredded, looking much like crabmeat.

There are 31 spinal nerves that branch off (front and back) from the spinal cord and thread their way through the openings between the vertebrae. If a disk is defective and protrudes even slightly, it can press a nerve. That's the rub—the nerve rub that causes backache, sciatica and even loss of feeling in toes.

You need to understand that disks have essentially two degrees of degeneration and protrusion to cause major and minor degrees of trouble. The first degree occurs when the fibrous skin of the disk starts to bulge like an auto tire at a weak spot. Sometimes it is so small that even when a surgeon opens up his patient's back and looks at the disk he can't detect the protrusion.

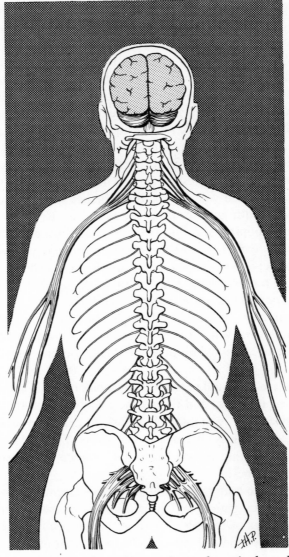

*Nerve trunkline. The spine conducts the spinal cord, the main trunkline of nerves from the brain to the organs and limbs of the body. Those that continue to the legs are called the sciatic nerves.     Fig. 3*

To use another food analogy, a degenerative disk is like a grape. If you start to squeeze a grape, you can exert pressure up to a level without breaking the skin. Then, if you stop squeezing and release the pressure, the grape will assume its previous round shape. However, if you don't let up on the pressure, the skin will break and the pulp will leak out. And you can never get those juicy contents back into the skin. The grape will never again be the same.

Thus with a degenerative disk. It will bulge with pressures; as pressures ease, the bulge will lessen. But if the pressures on it continue, the fibrous ring will rupture and allow the nuclear substance to escape. Because there is a tough, thick ligament pressed tight against the front of the vertebrae, the contents of a ruptured disk seldom leak forward. Instead they usually burst toward the back and protrude into the vertebral (spinal) canal there, pressing hard on the spinal cord or the spinal nerve roots.

You should understand that even when you are lying down and your back is at "rest," there are tremendous intervertebral pressures being exerted. This is the unfelt springlike action of the pair of shiny white ligaments that run down the entire length of the vertebral column—the thick one in front and a thinner one in back. There are also the shorter ligaments stretched in between adjoining vertebrae at the W-shaped bones.

When a disk ruptures, herniates, or "slips," its substance squeezes out with considerable force. (The three words describe essentially the same condition.) The resulting pressure on nerves usually causes severe pain in the back, which triggers the muscles of the back to go into spasm, nature's way of putting the back in a splint and thus immobilizing it to minimize the pressures on nerves. The disks that most normally rupture are those between L5 and S1 and between L4 and L5, which is where nerves to the legs branch off from the spinal cord. That is why sciatica—pain running down the back of the leg—is common in disk problems. Sometimes a nerve of sensation from a leg is also affected; the result can be anesthesia—or loss of feeling—of the foot or its toes. Sometimes, too, a herniated disk can cause disruption in functions of the organs of the abdomen. It can even cause impotence, bowel and bladder dysfunction, or paralysis, although these occur only rarely.

You can see, too, how people complain that they were "only raising a window," or "stooping to pick up something from the floor" when they "froze" in position. What happened was that as a result of improperly bending their backs (as we'll see later) they imposed tremendous pressures on an already weakened disk and "squeezed the grape" a bit too hard.

There is a very good reason that the lumbar disks, especially at L4 and L5, are the most frequent to herniate. The lumbar portion is like a fulcrum: all the motions of your upper spine pivot around it. And here is focused the weight of your head, shoulders, arms and chest. Thus, the lumbar region is subjected to forces that far exceed those to which all other parts of your backbone are subjected.

You probably consider most other people—those who do not have backaches—to be rather lucky. They are. They did all the things you did and yet *your* back is bothering you, while they feel fine. That should give you a clue to the fact that you were born with some sort of defect in your back. This defect may be a structural one or it may just as easily be some sort of predisposition. Perhaps there was a small malformation in the troublesome vertebrae or disk. Or perhaps one of these parts of your back had a weakness that was exploited by abuse or by some forgotten injury—perhaps a fall, kick or other blow you received as a child.

A study by Dr. John C. Wilson, Jr., of the University of Southern California, reported in 1969, suggests that herniated lumbar disks run in families. He found that many of his bad back patients had unusually thin, small disks that aged more rapidly than normal disks and that caused more problems than the thicker, bigger disks of patients who had no lower back problems.

If you've ever seen a human skeleton in a medical museum you probably noticed that its bones were wired together —even those of the spine. At the beginning of this chapter we said that your backbone is made of vertebrae that are stacked like a swaying pile of poker chips. That's too simple

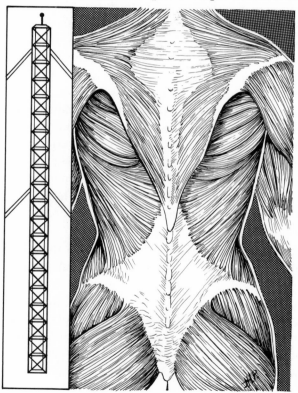

*Standing straight. Like the guy wires that hold up a radio mast (left), the muscles of the trunk can help hold up a weak or diseased spine (right).  Fig. 4*

an analogy, of course, but it does serve the purpose of telling you that the vertebral column has no inherent strength. By itself, it is just a stack of bones. That's why vertebrae of museum skeletons have to be wired together.

The ligaments of the spine that we just mentioned help keep vertebrae together as a unit and help to give them their springlike tension. But your spine is still happier lying than standing. What holds it up are muscles. Think of your spine as a tall television tower that has little inherent strength, but stands erect by a system of steel guy wires. Muscles and ligaments, together, are the guys of your spine.

One important set of muscles is obvious: those of your back. These are not as individually distinguishable as the muscles of your arms and legs—such as the *biceps* and the *rectus femoris*. Instead your back muscles are a system of closely knit tissues. Going from outer to inner, these extend the length of your back, then become more separate and shorter, until single muscles attach to each vertebrae. Spread over the back muscles are the larger muscles of the shoulders (such as the *latissimus dorsi*) and the larger muscles of the legs (the *gluteus maximus* that you sit on). These muscles use the spine as a foundation to pull against in order to achieve motion and to do work.

The muscles of the back that run parallel to the spine are those that hold it erect. If you straighten your spine out, you can reach behind with your hand and feel these muscles contract. This action is called the *extension* of the spine. Normally, the deeper layers of these muscles work without your thinking of them. But they can get weak and then they need to be strengthened through exercise, a subject we'll talk about in detail in Chapter 10. From head to hips, the average person can lean back and create an angle of 115 degrees. Carnival contortionists can achieve 260 degrees!

There is another set of muscles that control your back, although you may not have considered them in this way. They are your abdominal muscles, particularly those called the *rectus abdominis*. Tighten your tummy and you feel them contract—unless you're too flabby. When you lie in bed on your side and curl up into the fetal position, this is called *flexion*. Those abdominal muscles achieve this for you.

Along your sides are other sets of muscles. One is the *obliques,* which run along your ribs. Under your armpits are the *latissimus dorsi,* the muscles that rotate your trunk as they hold up your spine.

So now you see that the stack of bones called vertebrae is held vertical (as viewed directly from front or back) by all of the muscles of your trunk working together. If one set of muscles is allowed to weaken through disuse or becomes weak as the result of disease, the other muscles will work to pull the spine out of its proper shape. The S-curve of your spine may also be askew because your posture has become sloppy. This, too, can be corrected by exercise and by learning proper body mechanics, which, again, will be discussed in detail later in the book.

This short course in anatomy of the back was necessary if you are to understand your backache and what you can do and what your doctor can do—or cannot do—to alleviate it. If it has achieved its purpose, this primer has given you an appreciation of the factors that make your loins (i.e., your lumbar area) hurt. Now let's put it together and give you an idea of what slipped disk, sprains, slipped vertebrae and arthritis are all about.

To paraphrase Shakespeare, the fault is not in our stars but in ourselves. You may have a disk between your lumbar vertebrae that is not as thick or as full as it ought to be. You could get away with such a minor defect elsewhere along your spine, but here on the lumbar portion rests all the weight of your trunk, your shoulders and your head. Being an erect animal begins at the lumbar spine.

You sleep on a soft mattress and on your stomach. You don't exercise as often or as intensively as you should, and (whether you sit or stand all day) you have sloppy posture. You hunch over a lot and let your pot belly protrude. And when you lift, you bend over at the waist and use only your once-strong arms. The result of all this is that your lumbar vertebrae are almost always flexed—curved to the back instead of forward. Or perhaps your stomach has become so soft and so big that you have become swaybacked, like an old horse. In either situation, you impose tremendous pressures on your vertebrae—pressures that make the disk's life difficult.

If a disk is faulty, its insides start squeezing out like toothpaste from a tube. You feel a twinge and a pain now and then, but you pay no special attention to it. After all, you're getting older, aren't you? Pains, especially in the back, are to be expected every once in a while, aren't they? Then one day, when you least expect it, it hits. You may be brushing your teeth, opening a window, hitting a golf ball (as in Ted's case), bending to pick something up or twisting to reach for a ball during a tennis match when you freeze. The pain is so intense you can't move. The insides of the disk have popped. They have burst out and slammed against your spinal column, inflaming a nerve. Suddenly your entire back stiffens and you literally cannot move; if you try to, it feels as though a hundred needles are pricking your back. You may simultaneously feel a hot, burning pain behind your thigh. You have to be carried, or at least helped, to a doctor.

Even without a bad disk, your back may go into spasm. It could be that you have truly sprained or strained your back muscles. Again, if you do not exercise regularly and keep in good shape all those guy muscles that hold you erect, you are susceptible to this kind of injury. When you strain a muscle, you apply an unusual force and catch it off guard. When you suffer a sprain, you apply a force when the muscle is in an awkward, absolutely abnormal position. In either case, tissues are stretched beyond normal and the result is injury (often tearing) of muscle, tendons and nerves.

It sounds simple enough, but what often happens is that you don't seek help or don't rest your back and the condition becomes chronic. What happens then is that the muscles of the trunk get into a new relationship of pulling and tugging and you are set up for a long period of backache.

If those vertical spurs of bone of the vertebrae—the articular processes—don't meet properly and you have that condition known as *spondylolysis,* you have still another condition that can upset the muscle balance. If you do not sleep, sit and stand properly, and do not exercise the proper muscles, the weak vertebra can slip forward. Slipped vertebra is the very serious condition known as *spondylolisthesis,* in which the entire spine is thrown out of line and must be immediately operated upon.

If you have some arthritis of the spine, there will be pain sometimes because of the irritation of the bones and the vertebral joints. Again, if your trunk muscles are not in proper tone and you are not careful, the pain of the condition can pull the wrong muscles at the wrong time, worsening the condition as well as your pain.

Some doctors believe that taller people are more likely to have back trouble than are shorter people. Experts look at the dachshund whose (often bad) back is proportionately longer than its legs, and say that, likewise, taller people have disproportionately longer spines, yet the same number of vertebrae. Therefore the angular movement—and consequently, pressures on the disks—are greater. Also, the taller person's ligaments, tendons and muscles are stretched longer and so are more susceptible to injury than the shorter person's.

So far this is a theory, not proved. After all, height is not necessarily linked to spine length. Many people are tall or short because of the length or shortness of their legs.

Height was one of the identifiable factors cited by Dr. Joseph Tauber, the physician in charge of employees at the Jones & Laughlin steel plant in Aliquippa, Pennsylvania, in his study of backaches. His report on backache factors appeared in the April, 1970, issue of the *Journal of Occupational Medicine*. He found that 46 per cent of the backache cases were men 5 feet 11 inches or taller—whereas only 15 percent of the average male population was that tall.

In his study of 737 cases during four years, he found that the highest frequency of backaches occurred during warm months, with September being the month of greatest backache incidence. August, May and July were runners-up.

The idea that aging is a factor was not borne out in Dr. Tauber's study. He found that workers in the 18- to 24-year age group had consistently higher rates of backache than other age groups: the 25- to 34-year group was next.

Dr. Tauber concluded with this statement as to why so many of his backache cases were younger men: "Just as erect walking has to be learned, so must work, with the involvement of the back and the tolerance to backaches."

# 3. That Ache in Your Back

The purpose of this book is to help you to understand and to learn how to successfully live with that ache in your back. One of the first things you need to get clear is that there are many different causes of pain in that area of your back approximately between your ribs and pelvis. You probably think that what hurts is your spine, that you suffer from a "bad back." You may be right, but the spine is just one of the structures and organs in that part of your body; any of these can give you a backache.

It is essential that before you go any further in this book, you are sure that the source of your backache is not something else and somewhere else. That's a good reason to be under a doctor's care. Don't diagnose your backache. Your doctor may tell you that the pain comes *not* from the spine and back muscles. If that is the case, this book is not for you. That many diseases and conditions can masquerade as back pain has been known since the era of ancient Greece, when Hippocrates (the father of modern medicine) wrote, "Illnesses starting with pain in the back run a difficult course."

One of the reasons for his statement is that vital organs are located in this general area, and if they became diseased (especially at that time before antibiotics, artificial kidneys and other such contributions of modern science to medicine), the consequences could be longterm and dire.

The rest of this chapter will explain the many causes of backache so that you can have a proper perspective of your problem. What follows is an outline of backache causes listed in eleven general categories from A (arthritis) to T (tumor). Please keep in mind that these are the most general causes. There are many other specific and exotic sources of backache that are not common enough to be of any importance to you. After all, this is not a textbook for doctors, but a guide for back sufferers like you.

1. ARTHRITIS. There are two kinds relevant here: degenerative and inflammatory.

*Degenerative arthritis* is also called osteoarthritis. Simply stated, it is the result of wear and tear on your joints. Your spine—as we've explained in the previous chapter—is an S-curved line-up of bones (called vertebrae), which move, like most other bones, by sliding on their neighbors at junctions called joints. The surfaces of adjoining bones that meet in a joint are normally covered with smooth, elastic and slippery cartilage. While the exact cause of osteoarthritis is unknown, it seems to come with aging and so you're bound to get a touch of it in some joint or another if you live long enough. What happens is that the cartilage becomes pitted and frayed and may deteriorate until it is completely worn. The rubbing bones thicken and sometimes they develop little spurs that hinder movement even more. Then the ligaments and muscles of the back that move these bones of the spine go out of balance and become tense, causing pain. Sometimes, the bony spurs press on nerves and cause pain directly. There is nothing at all new about osteoarthritis of the spine. It has been identified in such prehistoric remains of humans as Java man and Neanderthal man, in mummies from ancient Egypt and in skeletons unearthed from pre-Columbian mounds in the New World.

Three kinds of *inflammatory arthritis* cause backache. One is rheumatoid arthritis, which is the most dangerous, destructive and disabling form of arthritis. It hits three times as many women as men and can attack the spine as it does any of the joints of the body. Sometimes it hits suddenly, but more often it creeps up subtly and insidiously with aches and pains that last a few days and disappear, only to reappear with more intensity. Eventually it becomes a daily problem that cannot be ignored. The spine is not the most common site attacked by rheumatoid arthritis, but since the disease often affects the whole body, it can be. When rheumatoid arthritis invades a joint, the joint becomes stiff, swollen and tender, making motion painful and difficult. It is usually worse in the morning than in the afternoon. Unchecked, it can destroy the joint, cause the connecting bones to fuse and become immobile. While this deterioration of the joint progresses, the muscles pull it into a grotesque shape.

*Ankylosing spondylitis* is similar to rheumatoid arthritis. However, its victims differ: it attacks men ten times more frequently than women, and almost always when they are young adults. Also called Marie-Strümpell disease, it causes a fusing of the bones of the spine until it is rigid. But the stiff spine is not always straight; it can "freeze" in a permanent stooping curve. It specifically occurs in the lower back and one of the first signs is pain there and in the legs. After a few years, the disease goes as suddenly as it came, leaving the fused vertebrae in its wake, which on X-ray look like a shaft of bamboo.

*Gout* is a special form of arthritis which comes not (as legend says) from port wine and good living, but from a defect in body chemistry that its unhappy victims are born with. The problem is that the body contains more uric acid (a normal body substance) than the kidneys can get rid of. As a result, excess uric acid accumulates as needlelike crystals in joints, provoking inflammation. The inflamed joints—three out of four times the big toe is affected first—become hot, swollen and exquisitely tender. The joints of the spine can also be affected. There are good medicines (colchicine is foremost) to counter the attack of gout, and other medicines (probenecid and allopurinol) to help the body get rid of more uric acid, but prevention is also a key to its control. Gouty patients should eat diets that are at the same time low in purine and adequate in fluid, such as milk, egg, cheese, and bread, avoiding high-purine foods such as sweetbreads, liver, kidney, brain, gravy, and sardines.

2. CONGENITAL. If you develop arthritis of one form or another, or a bad disk, it is in part because you have an inherited disposition to the disease; you were not born with it, but are more susceptible to it than other people. Also, there are some other causes of backache that are congenital or present at birth. The most common one is a "slipped vertebra," due to a failure of proper connection and positioning of adjoining vertebrae because of the way the bones are formed or misformed. As a result, one vertebra slips ahead of the other, causing undue pressures. The less serious form of the condition, and perhaps a precursor of the more serious type, is called spondylolysis. This is very difficult to diagnose, except by X-ray, where in oblique view it casts a shadow that actually looks like the head and front paws of a Scotty dog or terrier. The more serious and permanent form is called spondylolisthesis. Twice as many men as women suffer from spondylolisthesis, which sometimes starts causing low back pain in childhood, but more often begins to pain in young adulthood. When a vertebra "slips," weight is imposed on the spine unequally, causing strains and sprains on the muscles and causing the growth of fibrous scar tissue that can rub on nerves and add to the pain.

3. DISK. Since most of this book will deal with problems of intervertebral disks, we won't go into much detail here. The disks, as we've explained, are the cushions between the vertebrae. When they protrude or rupture or develop other problems, they can impose on nerves and produce pain that leads to muscle spasm and the inability to stand, sit or work.

4. EMOTIONAL. The back is one of the body's emotional weather vanes, another way in which your mind or emotions or psyche lets you know something isn't right with you. Your back is a very psychosomatic area. In medical terms, back pain is often a somatic (physical) expression of a psychic disorder. Sometimes, too, your emotions can intensify the pain caused by a disease condition in your spine or elsewhere. Sometimes it superimposes an additional pain. Other times, it can bring on pain by itself; and emotionally caused pains are just as real as those brought on by irritated nerves. Such back pains can be considered messages that your psychological self is sending to your physical self. To cite a real example, when some women are hostile to their husbands and resent the thought of having sex with them, their minds cause their backs to hurt. The sex act only intensifies their back pain. The pain is quite real, but its source is not in the back but inside the skull. Using the same area of human activity—sex—some men who are latent homosexuals—and therefore impotent with members of the opposite sex—may develop backache as a psychological mechanism to keep them from having heterosexual relations. Backache can also be a sign of problems at the shop or office.

5. INFECTION. A report appeared in the January 4, 1971, issue of the *Journal of the American Medical Association* (pp. 113-115) describing the case of a 49-year-old woman who first suffered lower back pain in 1954, and had a series of hospitalizations. In April, 1969, she went to the Mayo Clinic with a skin rash, fever and low back pain. She was given an extensive battery of tests. The results convinced

the Mayo doctors that an operation was necessary. But let them tell it: "The lumbar wound was exposed. When the deep fascia was incised, a copious amount of thick green pus came forth. The abscess had surrounded the laminae and spinous processes of the lower three lumbar vertebrae. The cavity of the abscess was excised. . . ." The lab reported that the pus was the product of one of the most dreaded kinds of bacteria: Golden staph, more properly known as *Staphylococcus aureus*. The surgeons cleaned the pus out and gave the patient an antibiotic. Twelve days later they closed the skin, and put in plastic drains, through which they periodically washed out the wound. Twenty-two days after the pus-discovering operation, her skin rash disappeared. A week later she was allowed to walk. Thirty-eight days after her spinal abscess was discovered, she was discharged from the hospital.

The reason for telling you the gory details of this case is not to shock you, but to make you aware of the fact that infections can cause chronic low back pain. Staph is just one kind of bacterium that can infect the low back. Others are streptococci, gonococci, pneumococci, and meningococci—the germs that cause strep, gonorrhea, pneumonia and meningitis. Syphilis is another, caused by *Treponema pallidum*. Before the discovery and application of such antibiotics as penicillin, streptomycin and aureomycin, these infections could not only cause pain, but also severely cripple their victims by deforming the spine. The germs would eat up the disks, then attack the bone, causing the vertebrae to permanently fuse. Such bone infections are generally termed *osteomyelitis*.

The most prevalent kind of spinal infection was caused by tuberculosis, and while no longer of epidemic proportion in the United States, it is still prevalent wherever malnutrition and crowding coexist. Tuberculosis of the vertebrae is sometimes called Pott's disease, after Percival Pott who first described it in English at about the time the United States was born (1779), which also was a time that tuberculosis was rampant throughout England and Europe. It took another century to identify the infectious agent: Robert Koch isolated the tubercle bacillus in 1882. It was yet another sixty or so years before the discovery of streptomycin, the first medicine to directly combat this bacterium.

Tuberculosis affects the spine after entering the body elsewhere, usually through the windpipe and lungs. Most often TB affects children between the ages of two and five years, but it also affects adults. You can have a latent TB infection for years before it breaks out. Usually the bacteria set up their spinal infections inside a vertebra, captured there by the capillaries of newly formed bone. Sometimes the infection is contained by a wall of calcium set up by the growing bone. But more commonly the infection eats up the vertebra and the disks above and below, and then the infection spreads to the neighboring disks. Often, too, the TB germs set up an abscess, in which they wreak heavy destruction in one area.

The first symptom of *tuberculous spondylitis* is pain. Another is a bulge in the skin over the spine. The back muscles are usually in spasm; there is often limping and the back is too straight.

Undulant fever, not too common in the United States anymore, can also cause low back pain. Its germ, called brucella, is spread to people from sick cattle, hogs and goats—usually from their milk. The tetracycline antibiotics are effective in defeating the brucellosis infection.

Another kind of infection that causes low back pain is fungus. Blastomycosis is one version that is widespread in America. This germ, akin to yeast, affects mostly young and middle-aged men. By the time it shows itself by bumps on the skin, it has wrought damage in bones—including those of the back—similar to the damage caused by TB.

Fortunately, there are new medicines against the blastomyces invaders; but they must be administered with great care by a doctor. One is hydroxystilbamidine; another is amphotericin B.

Another fungus infection that can infest the vertebrae is *Coccidioides immitus,* which is common in the soil of southern California and Central America. Its infection is technically called coccidioidomycosis, popularly San Joaquin fever, valley fever and desert rheumatism. This highly infectious fungus is carried by dust. Usually it causes a rash and runs its course in a week or two, but it can linger on and invade the vertebrae, as well as other parts of the body. Sometimes the infection occurs years after the fungus is contracted. Amphotericin B is the only medicine known to be effective against it at this writing.

Less common as a cause of back pain is the fungal infection known as actinomycosis, lumpy jaw, or ray fungus. Most often it infects young men. Fortunately sulfas and penicillin are effective against it.

Viruses are yet another kind of infection that produces low back pain. Probably the most common is shingles, or *herpes zoster,* which is caused by a virus that is brother to chickenpox. Shingles most often occurs in early summer and late autumn and most frequently affects people who are more than 50-years-old. The infection starts in a root ganglia in the spine and follows a nerve horizontally along the back and around the side. Usually the nerves of sensation infected are those along ribs, but it can occur lower down. The path of pain can precede by weeks the occurrence of a line of skin blisters. There is no effective treatment for the infection, which must be allowed to run its course. However, there is prevention: people who have had chickenpox and are still immune to it also seem to be immune to this virus.

6. INJURY. It should be obvious, but we'll state it anyway: if you have received a blow to your back, it will hurt. Thus, if you are the victim of an automobile or motorcycle accident, or if you have been thrown by a horse, or if you slip on ice, your back may be injured far more seriously than

you suspect. It doesn't take too much violence to fracture a vertebra. In other words, you can break your back by jumping from too great a height, even if you land squarely on your feet, or by falling while skating. Dive into too-shallow water and hit bottom, and you can break a vertebra. Sometimes a blow to the head can do it.

Fractures of the spine are more common in older people, whose bones have degenerated as part of the condition known as *osteoporosis,* in which the bones become depleted of calcium. Osteoporosis can also be the result of tumors of the adrenal or pituitary glands.

7. KIDNEY DISORDERS. Your kidneys are located approximately behind your floating ribs in the small of your back. So if they are diseased or disturbed, they can cause pain that you feel in your back. An infection of the kidney, kidney stones, tumor of the kidney, injury to the kidney or its reaction to certain drugs (such as mercurials) can be the cause.

To differentiate back trouble from kidney trouble, your doctor may do a Murphy's punch. Don't be alarmed if he does; it is for diagnosis only. This is a broad punch with the fist to the kidney area of the back. If your pain is intense, its source may be the kidney and not the back.

8. METABOLIC. We explained above (No. 6) that metabolic disorders caused by tumors of the adrenal and pituitary glands can weaken vertebrae by leaching out calcium and making them susceptible to fracture and, therefore, pain. Another glandular disorder can cause a similar condition. This is the oversecretion of the hormone of the parathyroid glands, which sit atop the thyroid glands in your neck. The hormone from these pea-sized glands regulates (among other things) the metabolism of calcium. It is a powerful agent to deposit calcium in or withdraw it from bone. When the gland oversecretes, calcium is withdrawn from the bone. Depleted of their calcium, bones (including vertebrae) weaken and break easily.

After menopause, women's bodies lack the sex hormones that in youth have kept their bones strong. This is true of some men too. Treatment with suitable hormone—estrogen or testosterone—can bring immediate relief to backache so caused.

Vitamin D deficiency (rickets) can also weaken bones and cause backache.

Paget's disease, which most often affects middle-aged men, causes changes to form in bones, including vertebrae. Its cause is unknown and the pain seems to leave as mysteriously as it comes, but in the meantime it can damage the spine and cause low back pain, and the bone change persists. Occasionally there can be a malignant change in this type of bone disease.

9. PREGNANCY. As the unborn baby grows in her womb, the pregnant woman's body's center of gravity shifts. It moves forward, actually stretching the spine and increasing its curve. This pull on the spine often causes backache.

Other changes occur in the body of the pregnant woman, which can make her back hurt. The hormonal output of her glands changes and causes corresponding changes in her bones and ligaments. Since this happens at a time when there is extra weight on her pelvis, these bones and ligaments stretch, often pulling on nerve fibers and causing low back pain.

Finally, labor itself often begins as a lower back pain— but one that comes and goes at regular intervals of five to ten minutes initially.

10. REFERRED PAIN. The pain of labor (just described) is a referred pain—one originating somewhere else in the body but felt in the back. Some women who have painful menstruation feel it not as abdominal cramps but instead as low backache. Furthermore, inflammations and infections of the uterus can cause backache.

In men, backache can be a referred pain from an infected

or inflamed prostate gland, as well as from an inflamed bladder.

In both men and women, backache can also be the result of disorders of some organ of the abdomen—including colitis, intestinal infections, appendicitis and duodenal or gastric ulcer (see *Living with Your Ulcer,* another book in this series). In some cases pernicious anemia can also cause backache.

11. TUMOR. A growth, especially a malignant growth, is certainly the most dire cause of backache. Because vertebrae are spongy and have such a rich blood supply, they are more likely than many other bones to capture seed cells cast off from a primary cancer elsewhere in the body, such as in the breast, uterus, prostate or lung. Such secondary cancers, called *metastases*, cripple and kill just as certainly as do primary cancers. At least half of the cases of cancers of the spine are caused by metastases. The rest are cancers and other growths that originate in the vertebrae, among which carcinoma is the most dreaded and perhaps most frequent. There are also benign growths of the vertebrae, such as giant-cell tumors.

In any case, growths cause back pain by invading healthy tissue and pressing on microscopic nerve endings. Particularly ominous is back pain in people over 40 years that gets worse at night.

As we said at the beginning of this chapter, our purpose is not to frighten you or to parade a list of pathological cases before you. Instead it is to help you understand that your back is indeed part of you—a vital, necessary and exceedingly responsive part of you. If you've taken it for granted until now, you won't any longer. When it hurts it is telling you something. The important thing for you to do is heed that warning and go to a doctor so he can find out what is the matter. Then, as you now appreciate, the doctor may have quite a chore to diagnose your condition and determine the specific cause of your pain.

# 4. How the Doctor Diagnoses Your Back Trouble

Your back is killing you. The pain and stiffness are major and legitimate symptoms. As you mention them to other people, you may find that those who have had back trouble empathize with you. But those who never had backaches may look at you differently. Some may even think you are malingering, faking or otherwise trying to fool them. This is particularly true if your back trouble started on the job or during some chore around the house.

Don't be overwhelmed by the feelings and emotional reactions you'll get about your back trouble. In previous times bad back was scorned as a weakness that only females and old people exhibited. It was called lumbago and "my rheumatism," or "the rheumatiz." People who have escaped it are still liable to be derisive.

Folklore coupled with the many possible causes of bad back make it one of the most difficult of man's ills to diagnose. Dr. Philip Wiles, a London orthopedic surgeon, expressed it well when he wrote:

Low back pain is one of the most common complaints met in

38

practice and its causes are so diverse as to make systematic description more than difficult. The symptoms have little variety, physical signs are few, radiological findings are equivocal, and pathological information is sketchy. There is little agreement as to the etiology, which is often speculative, and, as to treatment, which is usually empirical. . . . Medical men, for so long without any idea as to the real pathology of low back pain, jumped at the notion of a "slipped disk" as a gift from heaven, and many of them have exploited it to such effect that both they and the public have come to regard it as synonymous with low back pain. This is, of course, nonsense . . . the patient should be looked at as a whole. . . . There is no panacea for backache. Successful treatment is based on the painstaking consideration of the individual patient.[1]

As you read in Chapter 3, the list of causes of low back pain is long. Your doctor is not likely to discuss your condition as "slipped disk" or anything else without examining you thoroughly and running you through a battery of necessary tests. And if he can't be sure of your problem without a great deal of investigation, then neither can you! The worst thing you can do is to diagnose your condition, to try and treat it yourself, and/or to label it.

If you are smart, you'll call your family doctor and tell him what the trouble is as soon as your back hurts. Doctors use a great deal of art, even in this age of space exploration. Modern medicine is the artful use of science. You can't be its beneficiary unless you place yourself in a doctor's care (either your family doctor or an orthopedic specialist). When you do, he goes to work like a detective, using systematic investigation, using his personal powers of observation, using all the scientific diagnostic tools at his command. The object of his search is the "offender" that is causing your pain and stiffness.

[1]Philip Wiles, *Essentials of Orthopaedics* (Boston: Little, Brown, 1959), p. 52.

Your doctor will conduct much of the sleuthing in his office, but it is more than likely that he will also ask you go to the hospital for more detailed technical studies. If he suspects that you need immediate treatment, he will want you to be admitted promptly. In some instances, surgery needs to be performed without delay, as in some fractures and certain unremitting nerve pressures.

As a disease detective, your doctor will take nothing for granted. He will seek and examine all the evidence he can before he draws any conclusion or makes any diagnosis. And to come to a diagnosis, he has to eliminate all possible causes until he finds the most probable cause.

He will ask you questions—even questions you feel have no relevance—perhaps about your life-style, about your family and about your work. There are other times, too, when he will say nothing and perhaps make you uneasy and self-conscious because he is silently concentrating on you. Most of this observation will be while you are undressed, which may make you even more self-conscious. So might the fact that he will physically handle you more than he ever did before. There is no need for you to be uneasy. Just remember, it's your back he is interested in; to examine it properly he has to manipulate your limbs and your trunk. He can't observe these when they are covered.

It may seem maddening and unnecessary when you are in such pain, but unless there is a true emergency, your family doctor (or the specialist to whom he refers you) will want the answers to many questions. He will want to know about your general health, about the incidence of back troubles in your family, and about your history of falls, injuries, infections and other diseases. These would seem far-fetched questions if you did not have the background of the previous chapter and were not aware of the many possible causes of low back pain. So you should not be surprised if your doctor asks you about childbirth or prostate trouble—whichever is pertinent to your sex.

Your doctor will also question you in great detail about your back pain. He will want to know when it first occurred and he may press you to remember the very first time in your life that your back hurt. In-depth studies, mostly done in England during World War II, have shown that back troubles go back farther in a person's life than he usually remembers. Unrelenting inquiry will usually reveal you had a long history of back trouble, of repeated attacks with remissions or quiet periods of months and years. The pain may have even shifted from one side to another between attacks. Often the first pain can be linked to an athletic game you played in your youth or to a long-forgotten fall. Your doctor's questioning may remind you of the "click" or "crick" you once felt in your back, perhaps as you were working or playing ball.

The doctor will ask whether coughing, sneezing or moving your bowels affects your pain. He will ask you to describe the pain and try to locate its position. He'll want to know if the pain is only in your back or if it radiates to your legs (sciatica); if you feel any numbness; how the pain is affected by standing, sitting, bending, lying. As you talk, the doctor will note how you speak—especially if you talk when breathing in, as well as when breathing out, and whether you grunt as you speak.

After he has questioned you and talked to you (in medical terms, this is "taking your history"), the doctor will examine you. As we said, this will mean you will have to undress at least to your underwear in the privacy of the examining room. He'll observe the effects of pain as you undress. Then he'll ask you to stand as still and as erect as you can. As you do so, the doctor will note if you list to one side, if your shoulders are level, if your lumbar curve has straightened or if it is swaybacked. He may ask you to move your trunk to one side and then the other, or to rotate it. This is to assess the degree of any muscle spasm. He may ask you to try to touch your toes.

Then the doctor will ask you to get on to the examination

table. How you do so, and your facial expression, will tell much about the severity of your pain and about your limitation of motion. You may be asked to do sit-ups, with your knees either straight or bent. This is to assess ankylosis, and any tightness of the hamstring muscles at the back of your thighs.

Next, as you lie flat on your back, the doctor may ask you to keep your knees stiff as he raises first one leg, then the other. This is called the *Lasègue test*. Normally, you should be able to raise a leg an angle of 90 degrees or more. The test is positive if the pain is so intense that you can't allow the doctor to raise it that high. With the leg raised as high as it will go, the doctor may *dorsiflex* your foot, or manipulate it so the toes move toward your knee. This modification is known as *Bragard's test,* or the *sciatic stretch test.*

Some doctors are opposed to the use of the straight leg raise and the foot flex because these movements irritate the sciatic nerve. These doctors maintain that such irritation can increase the pain and worsen the condition. The irritation comes from the great squeeze forces imposed on the vertebrae and nerve roots with these leg-foot movements.

For this and for other reasons, your doctor may raise one of your legs, or both, with the knee(s) bent. He may also rotate both your raised bent legs: first to one side and then to the other. The purpose is to pinpoint the source of pain on the lower spine (sacroiliac or hip).

When the heel of one foot is placed on the opposite knee and then the raised leg and knee are pressed to the table, it is known as *FABERE-Patrick's test,* and is used to pinpoint the pain source to either hip joint or sacroiliac joint. If the knee cannot be pressed down very far, this can be the sign of 4, because that is the configuration the legs make. (FABERE is an acronym for Flexion, Abduction, External Rotation and Extension—the motions through which the legs are placed.) *Laguerre's test* is a variation in which the leg is placed into the same configuration but the heel is above and not touching the opposite knee.

There are several tests your doctor may perform while you lie on your side. One of the most common is *Ober's test,* in which you bend the leg that is under you, while the doctor presses on your hip with one hand; holding your free leg by the ankle, he rotates the leg and then lowers it to the table. This is to pinpoint pain in the sacroiliac joint and to detect any spasm or stiffness of muscles in the iliac crest just below your waist.

There are also tests he'll perform while you are prone, or lying face down. He'll place one hand on the small of your back and raise one of your legs by the ankle, with its knee bent. Called *Yeoman's test,* this stretches the ligament in front of the sacroiliac joint; normally the stretch produces no pain. However if your back hurts during the test, it rather specifically pinpoints the location of your trouble.

While you are still face down your doctor may also take hold of your ankles and bend the leg at the knee. This is called the *femoral nerve stretch test* or the *Ely test.* It pulls on the femoral nerve in front of the thigh in the same way as the sciatic stretch test pulls on that nerve at the rear of the thigh. If the femoral nerve test hurts, it may indicate irritation of the nerve roots at the third or fourth lumbar vertebrae.

In a third face-down test, your doctor will lift both of your legs off the table, with one hand across the front of your hips and one hand supporting your ankles. If this produces pain, it is an indication either of arthritis or of a minor muscle strain.

As we said, your doctor will be putting your legs and back through many unusual motions, in order to precisely locate the site of your pain. To do this, he has to handle you rather heavily. You can understand now why most orthopedists are so muscular and their handshakes so strong!

Your doctor may perform still other tests while you are on the examining table. For one thing, he may ask you first to sit on your heels and then to bend completely forward until your face is at your knees. With your spine thus fully flexed, he can locate tenderness and pain by merely pressing his fingers at different locations along your spine. He may in this way find a strained muscle or a "trigger point" from which pain is referred to other areas.

He will also take out his tape measure and see if your legs are the same length, and if your thighs and calf muscles are of the same diameters. He may ask you to get off the table and stand up as he places a small mark on the skin on each side of the site of the L3 or L4 vertebra, then stands a few feet away and observes. This is to determine if your pelvis is level. These measurements can give him clues to strain caused by uneven leg lengths. If the muscles of one leg are narrower than those of the other, this is a clue to disuse or favoring, usually the result of chronic pain, such as sciatica.

After he examines you, your doctor will no doubt send you to a radiologist to have X-rays made of your back. The radiologist may be located in a doctor's office building or in a hospital. In either case, it is best to go to this radiologist because your doctor can be certain of the quality of the X-rays he will then have to work with in the diagnosis of your bad back.

The X-ray can be very specific, as we said before, in the case of the "Scotty Dog" shadow of spondylolysis (explained in Chapter 3). Other times the X-ray is merely suggestive and highly subjective to interpretation.

The X-ray that is made is actually a film; in fact it is a black-and-white photographic negative. Unlike a usual photograph, however, this one is made with X-rays instead of with light. X-rays are just another form of electromagnetic radiation given off by electrons. Similar rays given off by natural substances (radioisotopes such as cobalt) are called gamma rays. Thanks to modern technology, X-rays are carefully produced so that the picture they produce for your doctor gives him the maximum information while you get the minimum dose. X-rays are invisible and unfelt as they penetrate your body. Bones are among the densest structures in your body; they hold back many of the rays and leave images on the film that are lightly exposed. Fleshy parts of your body, such as your skin and its underlying layer of fat, are transparent to X-rays and so the rays pass through readily and heavily expose the film. The result is that your body casts a shadowgraph on the film, with your vertebrae appearing white and your soft flesh appearing dark grey. The disks also appear dark since they are not opaque to X-rays as are the bones above and below them.

X-ray films of your back are not like black-and-white profile silhouettes of your vertebrae. The films are, in fact, shadowgraphs made of various lines and areas of different shades of gray. This means they can reveal the character of the surface of the vertebrae, as well as important details of the articular surfaces. The shades of gray can also reveal abnormal changes in the vertebral bone, such as osteoporosis and arthritis. In addition, the shadows can show and identify fractures of the vertebrae.

The X-ray can also indicate whether or not the vertebrae line up normally, or if one of the lumbar vertebrae has moved forward and out of place. The film will also clearly show the distances between the vertebrae. Too narrow a space between vertebrae can be an indication of an old slipped disk or disk injury.

You should clearly understand that the X-ray picture (often called a roentgenogram, in honor of the discoverer of X-rays, Wilhelm Röntgen) is at best a complicated shadowgraph that requires much interpretation. That is why both your own doctor and the radiologist (under whose direction the X-rays were taken) will study them and then consult about what they believe those images show. As the late Dr. Philip Lewin wrote, "The technic of making a roentgenogram is simple, but the interpretation may be difficult."

If your back is so painful and so incapacitating that your doctor sends you to the hospital, AND if he suspects that a disk has herniated, he will probably want you to have a myelogram taken. No test that is useful in diagnosis is perfect, but the myelograph is between 85 and 95 percent accurate. You have probably talked to other bad back patients —especially those who have been operated on—and heard all sorts of grim dire stories about myelograms. Here are the facts:

First of all you should understand that we are not talking about a myogram, which is a record of the contractions of muscle. A myelogram is a way to picture (graph) the spinal cord (myelo-). The spinal cord, your body's main trunkline of nerves, runs along your backbone from your brain to your tail. As we explained in Chapter 2, the spinal column's bony tunnel contains and protects the spinal cord. The nerves are enclosed for most of the length of your back in a long, thin casing, somewhat like some stretched-out sausage casing, which goes to the end of the spinal column. Inside the casing with the nerves is a watery liquid that circulates to and from the ventricles and subarachnoid space of the brain; this is the cerebrospinal fluid.

Pairs of nerves branch off from the spinal cord and run through intervertebral spaces at 31 points along your back. These nerve roots branch off with their own casings. The spinal cord ends at L1, the first lumbar vertebra, and the nerves, which extend lower, separate in a configuration known as *cauda equina* (horse's tail). The last (lowermost) five nerves come together again lower down (at about the height of your buttocks) to form that sometimes painful sciatic nerve, which runs down the back of each thigh.

Your myelograph will be performed in the hospital's X-ray department. You'll probably be prepared for the test with a tranquilizer about an hour or so before you are scheduled. You'll be taken to the X-ray room, where you'll be placed on the table on your side, with your knees bent. Local anesthetic will be injected into the small of your back to deaden it, and antiseptic will be washed on the area to prevent any infection. At the same time the X-ray tube will be lowered over you. Its dual purpose is to take X-ray films and to provide a continuous X-ray picture of your spine during the test. This is known as fluoroscopy.

Let us set some of your other fears to rest now, those about X-rays and fluoroscopes, because much has been said in the press about the dangers of fluoroscopy. In the early days of fluoroscopy, a screen was pressed against the near side of the body to capture the rays generated from the X-ray tube on the far side of the body. The X-rays made the screen glow and the dense parts of the body (like bone) appeared as moving shadows on the glowing screen. In the first days of X-ray at the beginning of this century, doctors were enthusiastic about its diagnostic uses but not aware of its potential dangers. They did not protect themselves from the rays; as a result, many developed cancer of the fingertips, leukemia and other fatal diseases. So fluoroscopy was pretty much abandoned as too dangerous.

Today however, fluoroscopes need but tiny amounts of X-ray to look inside you, thanks to television-like electronic devices that amplify the picture. Also, radiologists and orthopedists who work with fluoroscopes wear lead aprons and gloves to protect their bodies and hands.

As for you, you needn't be concerned about the doses of radiation you'll receive from medical X-rays. In the first place, if you are still of child-producing age, the doctor will probably shield your gonads with lead. In the case of X-rays of the lower back this is more readily done in men than in women because the testicles are far enough from the lumbar region; the ovaries of women are not. In the second place, you will not receive enough of a dose of X-rays to be dangerous. After all, you take such X-rays only a few times in your life. Radiologists, orthopedists and X-ray technicians are around as much X-ray in an hour as you will be in your lifetime.

There are two steps to the myelograph. The first is a spinal tap. This means the doctor will insert a long needle between two vertebrae. Chances are he will insert the needle between L2 and L3. He realizes your injured disk is probably lower, but he doesn't want to do anything that will worsen your condition. If you do have some disk material protruding rearward he doesn't want the needle to penetrate it and further bother nerves that are already irritated. Experience has shown that 80 percent of herniated disks are located at L5 and S1 and that 19 percent are at L4 and L5. Furthermore, he'll insert the needle under X-ray direction to be sure he is clearly between the vertebrae and to be certain of the depth of the needle: he wants it to just penetrate the myelin casing.

Once the needle is where he wants it, he will use the attached syringe to withdraw a sample of 150 drops, or 10 cc., of the clear liquid. This sample of spinal fluid will then be sent to the laboratory where it will be tested for protein content. A slight elevation of protein content indicates irritation; a large elevation can indicate a tumor or infection. Some of the fluid will also be placed under a microscope in a search for cells. White blood cells indicate infection or other disease.

The second phase is the making of the myelogram. Using the same needle, but another syringe, the doctor will squeeze into the spinal fluid around the cord a small amount of opaque substance known as Pantopaque. Chemically known as iophendylate, it is a thin, oily compound that contains iodine. Iodine, in the jargon of the profession, is radiopaque, which means it is opaque to X-rays, thus casting a sharp shadow on film.

The table you are on will be tilted until the Pantopaque flows to the exact intervertebral space your doctor suspects. If his suspicion is verified, the white column of Pantopaque will be indented on the screen at one spot by the protruding disk. This is circumstantial evidence of a slipped disk and is usually strong enough evidence to lead to surgery—when other signs point that same way.

While the Pantopaque is in your spinal cord, the radiologist will be pushing buttons and the apparatus below and above you will be making whirring, clicking, grinding sounds. Those are the sounds of X-ray films being taken. These films will be later studied in great detail by the radiologist and by your own doctor.

After the myelogram is complete, the Pantopaque will be sucked back through the needle. (This is not the current practice in Great Britain, however.) A small bandage will be placed over the puncture site, you'll be helped off the table onto a cart and returned to your room. You will probably be asked to lie flat in bed for 12 to 24 hours.

You should know that some people experience some nausea and/or headache after a myelogram. This discomfort can last anywhere from a day to a week; it usually represents the time it takes for your body to replace the cerebrospinal fluid that was removed in the puncture. Your doctor will give you medicine to help your discomfort, but it may linger even so. The degree of pain differs in different people: some say it is like a dull headache, while others say it feels as though the top of their head is coming off. And no philosophic words about the eventual relief of back pain can help at the time.

Two things need to be said about the iodine. If you are allergic or otherwise sensitive to this chemical element, you should tell your doctor in advance of the myelogram. We don't mean that when you put tincture of iodine on a cut or a

sore that it burns. Everyone feels that. We mean an allergy
to foods and medicines containing iodine as a component.

Also, iodine is intimately involved with the functioning
of your thyroid gland and its control of metabolism. There
isn't enough iodine left in your body to affect your metabolism, but there is enough to make wild the results of any
thyroid test you take. It usually takes many months for the
iodine to be cleared from your body. Keep that in mind if
sometime after your bad back hospitalization, you are sent
to have a thyroid test for one reason or another.

There are so many causes of low back pain, that your doctor is going to eliminate all other possibilities before he diagnoses your trouble as slipped disk—or whatever. Slight nar-
rowing of the disk space between vertebrae is not by itself a
sure reason for a diagnosis of slipped disk. No two backs are
alike; many of us have slight deviations from the so-called
normal as we develop, Myelograms are usually conclusive,
but not always. Sometimes the diagnosis is finally made only
on the operating table.

Your doctor will use every available test to arrive at a
diagnosis before then. In the hospital, samples of your blood
will be taken and sent to the lab for analysis; so will samples
of your urine. If your doctor suspects a kidney infection or
kidney irritation, he'll give you a Murphy's punch, as explained earlier in the book, and ask that your urine be cul-
tured, that is, placed in a microbiological culture to see if
any germs are present to grow.

Chapter 3 detailed the possible causes of low back pain
which your doctor will consider as possibilities. On the basis
of learning about the nature of your pain, and your history
of illnesses, and after having physically examined you and
seen your X-rays, he'll narrow down the possibilities by elim-
inating unlikely causes. Pains and malfunctions of other
parts of your body can give strong clues to pains and mal-
functioning of your lower back. For instance, a heart con-

dition known as cardiomyopathy has been linked with spondylitis; both can be the result of rheumatic fever. A man's inability to have an erection may be due to emotional causes, but it might also be due to massive rearward protrusion of the disk at L4/L5, particularly if it is coupled with bladder trouble and some paralysis of the leg or foot.

If your doctor suspects arthritis, he may order a test that detects specific protein (known as rheumatoid factor) in your blood. Gout can be confirmed by abnormally high levels of uric acid in your blood. An infection in your back can reveal itself by fever (even low-grade fever of just over 100°F.) and, more certainly, by germs in the area of the pain or even in the spinal fluid. These germs will be sent to the lab and grown in cultures for certain identification and for testing as to which antibiotics they are most susceptible.

Your doctor may order a radioisotope scan of your back. This means some strontium-85 would be injected into your body. Strontium is chemically close to calcium and, like calcium, is incorporated into new bone that is formed in such conditions as osteomyelitis, as well as in fractures, Paget's disease and even in cancer. Because the strontium-85 is radioactive, it imperceptively sends out small and harmless emissions of radiation that are detected by a machine called a scanner. The scanner will "see" more radiation where there is more strontium-85—at the disease site—and will display this as a concentration of dots on a scan picture of your back.

If you are a woman with past gynecological problems, your doctor may examine (or ask a gynecologist to examine) your vagina, uterus and ovaries and give you other tests (such as hormone determinations) to see if your low back pain is being referred from these "female organs" in your pelvis. If you are a man with previous prostate trouble or an enlarged prostate now, your doctor may want to give you further tests and examinations (or ask a urologist to do so) to see if this is the source of your back pain. Likewise, if you have had a stomach ulcer before, or if your doctor suspects you have one now, he will order X-ray tests of your stomach, and perhaps even a gastroscopic examination to look at the stomach directly. An active ulcer, particularly a posterior ulcer, may be causing the back pain. If you look pale or are underweight, your doctor may also order some blood tests, or even a blood marrow test (usually made by means of a needle into your breast bone) to see if you are anemic, and why.

As we said at the beginning of this chapter, your doctor is a disease detective. When you come to him complaining of a pain and maybe some stiffness in your back (and possibly in your legs), he'll begin an investigation as thorough as that of any Scotland Yard or FBI investigator on a criminal case. Your doctor will follow every lead and leave it only when it comes to a blind alley. Once he has all his data, your doctor will literally sit back and analyze them. First, he'll eliminate the improbable causes of your pain. Then he'll review the possible causes and finally narrow these down to the probable cause or two. Only then will he go on to the next phase: your treatment.

You should understand—as we said at the beginning—that medicine is the artful application of science to health. That means there are no clear-cut certainties about diagnosis. Sometimes the doctor won't know exactly what the cause of your problem is until he treats it. Usually, if you respond and get better, it was the right diagnosis; if your pain doesn't get better, it wasn't. But even this concept is too simple. Pains often go away by themselves; often, too, there is more than one reason for pain, so treating one cause won't end the pain. Sometimes the cause—say a disk protrusion—isn't discovered until surgery.

Treatment is the subject of the following three chapters. The next chapter tells about the nonsurgical treatment of back trouble in the hospital. If you know you are going to have a back operation, you can skip Chapter 5 and go on to Chapter 7, which describes back surgery.

## TABLE 1.  CLUES TO PRESSURES ON LOWER LUMBAR NERVE ROOTS

*L4 root (L3 or L4 disk):*
   Pain and numbness of back and side of thigh, across knee, and of front and side of lower leg.
   Weakness on extension of knee.
   Decreased knee jerk reflex.
   Shrinking of thigh muscles.

*L5 root (L4 disk):*
   Pain and numbness of front and side of lower leg and of top of foot and big toe.
   Weakness on the pulling up of foot and great toe.
   Shrinking of muscles of shin.

*S1 root (L5 disk):*
   Pain and numbness of back and side of lower leg and side and sole of foot.
   Weakness on pushing down of foot and great toe.
   Decreased or absent ankle jerk reflex.
   Shrinking of the calf muscle.

*Lumbar disk L4 and L5:*
   Pain in backs of both thigh and lower leg.
   Numbness of buttocks, between legs, backs of both thighs, legs, and soles of feet.
   Weakness (often paralysis) of feet and legs.
   Knee jerk reflexes are active, but ankle jerks are absent.
   Shrinking of both calves.
   Paralysis of bowel and bladder, with perhaps other symptoms.

# 5. Treating Your Back in the Hospital

Of course you don't like the idea of having to go to the hospital. It's quite a normal reaction. After all, it means separation from your family and friends. It means isolation from your usual surroundings and neighborhood. It means forced absence from your work and from your coworkers—and perhaps it means some loss of income. It means rearranging the family routine to allow for your absence, for care of the children and their meals, for visiting you in the hospital.

When your doctor tells you he wants you to go to the hospital, you may also be suddenly frightened by the thought that your bad back is more serious than you had realized. After all, only *really* sick people go to the hospital, you may believe, or people who are dying. Maybe, you think, your condition is far worse than your doctor is willing to tell you.

Even when you understand why your doctor wants you to go to the hospital (as you will after reading this chapter), you will have an emotional reaction when he tells you. That's only natural. You should understand that even doctors and medical writers (like the authors of this book) are concerned

and worried and anxious and somewhat fearful when told they must go to the hospital for treatment.

But they also realize, as you should, that hospitals are not dismal places only for the deathly ill. You should realize that they are places for healing and as pleasant as can be. Most bad back patients enter tilting or even horizontal, but leave vertical. They are in far more pain when they are helped into the hospital than when they walk out. Your doctor sends you to the hospital only because your back is bad enough that it needs the kind of skilled and continual attention it can get there.

Fear of hospitalization is one reason that too many bad back sufferers look for the "quick cure" so often promised by the patent medicine hucksters and quacks. You know from reading Chapter 3 that there are many causes of back pain and that there can thus be no universal "miracle medicine" to make all pain go away. Nor is there any other kind of "treatment" that works instantly to effect a permanent cure, be it heat, ultra-sound, manipulation or whatever.

There is just no quick cure or short-cut treatment of bad back. It took time to deteriorate and it will take time to heal. Further, it may never be cured. There is a good chance that your life will never again be totally the same, that you will have to change some of the things you do, at work and/or at play.

The best place for starting the treatment of a back that is in acute pain is in the hospital. Sometimes this means a surgical operation, which is the subject of Chapters 7 and 8. This chapter will deal with only the nonsurgical treatment of bad backs, as a continuation of the previous chapter, which explained how your doctor diagnosed the cause of your bad back, probably with tests performed in the hospital.

The length of your stay in the hospital will depend on the condition of your back and on how it responds to treatment. The average bad back patient needs to stay in the hospital for about ten days. But you should be prepared to stay for anywhere from three days to nine weeks. After your doctor makes his diagnosis, he will be able to estimate the length of your stay in the hospital. Just remember, though, that it is an estimate, not a guarantee. Where bad backs are concerned, there are no guarantees.

The primary reason for hospitalizing you is to put your back at rest. And your mind. Your back can never get better while you are physically and emotionally aggravating it. In the hospital, you will be confined to bed so as to physically prevent you from moving your back and from thus further irritating the muscles, tendons, bones or disk involved.

The hospital is a different world; it is a therapeutic environment in which you have no choice but to lie back and enjoy it, to let everyone around—nurses, aides, physical therapists, dietitians, doctors—take care of you. Thus you have nothing to worry about. Even the anxieties you may have about your family and your work somehow, after your first day of hospitalization, become remote from this hospital world.

In a way, your hospitalization is a return to the womb. It is a place of warmth and of comfort where all of your biological needs are taken care of and are anticipated. For this reason, your doctor may prohibit phone calls and strictly limit your visitors, at least for the first few days of your stay. It is a good idea for your spouse or parent or best friend to brief the rest of your family and your friends and ask them not to bother you for a while; then when they do call or visit you, they should converse so as to not disturb your calm and your retreat.

During your stay at the hospital, you may have some diagnostic tests taken (as explained in the previous chapter), but the entire program of treatment directed by your doctor will be aimed at (1) relieving the pain you are suffering; and (2) doing everything possible to quiet the irritation causing your backache. Depending on the cause of your lower back pain, you may be treated by medication, heat, manipulation, injection, traction, bracing or exercise—each alone or in combination with others. And, of course, rest. That's about the best treatment your back can have at this point.

The kind of rest your back needs is for you to lie in bed on your back (supine). In that way your back can completely relax, all of it—tendons, ligaments, muscles, disks. Then there is no effort needed for you to be a vertical land-walking animal. This relieves from your back the 150 foot-pounds (or so) of energy it must expend to keep you erect with every step you walk.

Lying flat on your back on a bed with a firm but not rigid mattress is almost the best way for it to relax. The very best way is for the bed to be bent into a gatched position, or Williams position, so that your back is flat against the top half of the mattress which is tilted up at an angle; and the bottom half of the mattress is bent back so that your legs bend at the knees around it. In this position, with knees and hips flexed, there is even less strain on your lower back than when your legs are stretched out straight.

Doctors estimate that 85 percent of their bad back patients recover with what they call "conservative therapy." That means doing very little except letting nature take its course. Bed rest is the most essential part of conservative therapy for bad back. But there are other ways your doctor may help nature.

For one thing, he may put you in traction: he will place around your hips a cloth belt to which cloth strips and ropes are attached. These ropes are then run through pulleys attached to the foot of your hospital bed, and metal or bag weights are attached.

The doctor may tell you that the main purpose of putting you in traction is to pull on those trunk muscles that are in spasm, in an effort to make them relax. He may say that the traction will "persuade" these muscles to "give up" the spasm. But you should know that it would take about ten times as much weight to do that as what he probably applies. Usually weights of 10 to 15 pounds are applied. To effectively break the muscles' spasm, he would have to apply weights of about a hundred pounds. That much weight would pull you off the foot of the bed or require a medieval stretch rack.

No, the real reason that traction is used is to keep you in bed and to keep you immobilized there. That's not cheating, if that's what you are now thinking. Keeping you quietly in bed *will* break the spasm and make those muscles relax.

There is yet another way to physically relax those muscles. That is with heat. Heat has the wonderful ability to make muscles relax and to increase the circulation of blood, thereby bettering nutrition of the tissues involved and, as a result, speeding their healing.

Heat may be applied in several different ways. In the old days, hot water bottles and hot packs were used, but these cool and have to be changed. Electric heating pads are seldom used in hospitals, mostly because of the danger of overheating and of electrical shock. This heat is also superficial, as is the heat of infrared lamps.

Deep heat is more commonly given in the hospital by machines. One such machine is the diathermy, which literally beams radio waves into your muscles to get them vibrating and thus heat them internally. Ultrasonic therapy does about the same thing, but instead of radiowaves uses the energy of sound frequencies that are far beyond those which we human beings can hear.

You have to remember that while heat treatments feel good and do good, they mostly treat only the symptoms of spasm and pain. Perhaps the exception is in the case of arthritis, where ultrasonic therapy may actually work to dissolve the bony spurs that cause the irritation, as some doctors claim. But even here, the treatment is limited and in no case, is it a cure.

If your back has been strained or sprained, or if you have a herniated disk or a slipped vertebra, the rest–heat treatment will act to intercede and help break the pain-spasm-pain cycle. This vicious cycle does your condition no good. The irritation of nerves in your back triggers your muscles to convulse into tight spasm. These may be the erector muscles along your spine, or some of the guy muscles in your lower trunk. The reflex tightening of these muscles causes the backache and often further irritates nerves . . . and so forth. The aim of treatment is to break in and interrupt the cycle. Making the muscles relax is one way. If the basic problem is torn ligaments, they will heal faster and better when they are relaxed. Then the treatment can be a cure. If the basic problem is arthritis, slipped disk or in the vertebral joint, then relaxing the muscles will mainly relieve your pain, but will also prevent worsening of the condition caused by the muscle spasm.

In the case specifically of strains and sprains of the back, massage may follow heat treatment. This is really just another way to "convince" your muscles to relax. It serves to increase the circulation of blood and to move the muscles that have been in tight spasm.

These methods of getting your muscles to relax—heat and massage—are usually administered not at your bed but in the hospital's physical therapy department. As in Ted's case in the first chapter, once a day you'll be taken from your bed and put on a cart and wheeled to P. T., where you will be placed on another bed for your heat and/or massage treatment.

At some time during your life with your backache, someone you know is going to recommend that you see an osteopath or chiropractor. So we might as well talk about them now, as we explain about another kind of treatment known as *manipulation.*

Manipulation literally means the use of hands; in the case of the back, it means using the hands to rotate and move the spine so as to effect beneficial changes in the muscles attached to it. Manipulation is practiced more widely in Great Britain than in the United States and so British-trained physicians are more likely to turn to manipulation techniques to treat bad backs than are American doctors. One of the most famous American medical physicians to use and teach manipulation for lower back pain was Dr. Philip Lewin of Chicago. He devoted a whole section of his very thorough 1943 medical text on backache to manipulation. In his book he wrote that every doctor should learn manipulative therapy, but cautioned that "it is a delicate procedure and the technic must be exact because errors are often disastrous."

It's important that you understand that. Not to be frightened of manipulation, but to give it a proper perspective. It is no panacea. It is no cure. There are no such words used for backs that are bad. And, as in other kinds of treatment, it is helpful for some types, but not for all.

If, for instance, the cause of your backache is a disk protrusion, manipulation could be the *coup de grâce* that makes the disk pop open and herniate, causing you major problems. Where the disk has already herniated and there is direct pressure on—and irritation of—nerve roots, manipulation can be dangerous. Dr. Philip Wiles, a London orthopedic surgeon who otherwise uses and advocates manipulation cautioned, "A number of people are known to have sustained severe damage to the cord as the direct result of ill-advised manipulation." That is why, he wrote, bad back patients must be thoroughly examined and the cause of their problem diagnosed. Manipulation, he said, should never be used when there is pressure on the spinal cord and disease of the vertebrae. Similarly, in the case of alignment problems (spondylolysis or spondylolisthesis), manipulation could worsen the condition.

As an intern at Los Angeles County Hospital, one of the authors (RGA) cared for a patient who was found to have a tumor of the spine as the cause of his backache. Yet he had just been treated by manipulation by a chiropractor. The "treatment" had cost him precious time during which the growth advanced.

Chiropractors and osteopaths are two kinds of health practitioners who use manipulation for treating all kinds of diseases, not just for back ailments. So you should understand something about them and their training.

Chiropractors are identified by the initials D.C. (for Doctor of Chiropractic) given by one of the United States' twelve schools of chiropractic—not one of which is accredited by any of the nation's recognized educational accrediting bodies. There are between 14,000 and 25,000 chiropractors in the country. Chiropractic was started in 1895 by Daniel David Palmer, a Davenport, Iowa, grocer and fish peddler. Palmer changed careers after reportedly curing a janitor's deafness by "adjusting" his spine. Chiropractors still use spinal adjustments to treat every disease. They also use vitamins, enemas, diathermy and electricity. In the opinion of the American Medical Association, chiropractic is a cult and its practitioners are largely quacks. As a result, states do not allow chiropractors to prescribe medication; the national government does not reimburse them for treatment of patients in Medicare or other federally sponsored medical programs.

Osteopaths are a far cry from chiropractors, although Palmer seemed to have adopted some of the techniques first advanced by Andrew Taylor Still, M.D., founder of osteopathy, about a century ago. In 1892 Dr. Still opened the first school of osteopathy at Kirksville, Missouri. As of 1971 six schools that granted the D.O. (Doctor of Osteopathy) degree were accredited by the American Osteopathic Association, and recognized by the U. S. Office of Education. America's

13,000 osteopaths are given medical commissions by the military and are paid as physicians under Medicare and other federal medical-payment systems. Furthermore, as of 1971, 46 states and the District of Columbia gave full physician and surgeon licenses to osteopaths. Finally, the American Medical Association has recognized that osteopathic training is largely equivalent to medical training. Thus American osteopathy has come a long way in a century. Osteopaths, once confined to practicing only in osteopathic hospitals, are now on the staffs of many medical hospitals as well.

Osteopathy was founded on Dr. Still's theory that the body can best fight disease and repair itself by achieving an inner equilibrium, or homeostasis; that man, because he stands upright without being designed to do so, has trouble maintaining inner equilibrium because of undue pressures on spinal nerves. The way to relieve these pressures, said Dr. Still, was for the spine to be manipulated. *An Introduction to Osteopathic Medicine,* published by the American Osteopathic Association, explains:

> Manipulative procedures, applied through specifically-directed corrective force, helps tense muscles, tendons, and connective tissues surrounding joints to relax. The increase in muscle-fiber length resulting from the relaxation eases the tension on the proprioceptors, thus reducing sensory bombardment to the spinal cord. Reduction of this bombardment, in turn, may allow the entire body to return to more normal, homeostatic levels and permit segmentally related visceral structures to repair themselves under more normal conditions.
>
> Osteopathic manipulative therapy is based upon specific diagnosis, indicated or contraindicated by the patient's specific condition. It is scientifically applied through the training and experience of skilled osteopathic physicians.

So we have come full circle to Dr. Lewin: manipulation is satisfactory in some back conditions, but dangerous in others. Each patient must therefore be examined and his condition diagnosed before manipulation can possibly be considered.

We haven't really told you anything yet about the technique of manipulation. Without going into great detail, here is some information that can serve you to better understand it, should your doctor prescribe this sort of treatment for you.

Essentially, manipulation is like the diagnostic exercises described in the previous chapter. These are designed to rotate and bend the spine at different vertebral levels. The object is to move the vertebrae and muscles in ways that they do not usually move. Often this causes a click you can feel and the therapist can hear. The click should not alarm you; it only means that a vertebral joint has been moved or a joint capsule has been stretched, as when you crack your knuckles. Manipulation is performed while all the involved muscles are relaxed. The chief benefit is to stretch shortened muscles and tendons, or those that are in spasm, or adhesions or scar tissue that tend to otherwise tighten. Manipulation is often performed with the patient under local anesthesia.

The most common manipulation for chronic low back pain is for the doctor or therapist to gently rotate your shoulders and hips in opposite directions. This is done while you are lying on your back or side, with your bottom leg extended and your upper leg bent at the knee.

To assure muscles being relaxed, manipulative therapy is often done following a heat treatment or a massage, which may eliminate the need for local anesthesia.

There is still another way to manipulate your back: by yourself with proper exercise, the subject of a later chapter.

While you are in the hospital, your doctor may prescribe any of a combination of medicines. Some are to ease your pain or the irritation, others are to allay your anxieties and still others are to chemically relax your spastic back muscles.

Among the strongest painkillers you may be given in the hospital are the narcotics. With much publicity about the abuse of drugs, too many hospital patients tend to forget that these drugs offer wonderful relief from pain when properly applied under medical supervision. And you should not be afraid that an injection of morphine to ease your pain will make you a dope addict. Addiction to any drug is far more complicated. For one thing, you have to have an emotional need for such dependence. Of course, if your doctor suspects you are that kind of personality he won't risk narcotics on you.

Among doctors and nurses, painkillers are known as analgesics. They are classified as strong and mild. The strong ones obviously are used for the more violent pains. The most effective of both categories are derived from natural narcotics —essentially opium—or their chemically made artificial substitutes.

Morphine, one of the strongest narcotics used in the hospital, is reserved for the worst pain because of its other reactions in the body. Among these are interference with breathing, dizziness, nausea and vomiting. It also can make you drowsy, but that's not so bad since you're in bed with not much to do anyway. Demerol and Mepadin (meperidine hydrochloride) and Dolophine (methadone hydrochloride) are synthetics similar to morphine, which can have the same reactions, but are less severe.

It is more likely that your doctor will prescribe painkillers that are mild analgesics. Among these the most commonly used are codeine and aspirin. Like morphine, codeine is derived from opium; unlike morphine, which is usually injected, codeine is usually taken by mouth. The most common complaint is that codeine constipates, but doctors have a saying that when a patient gets concerned with his bowel movements, he's starting to feel better. Aspirin is perhaps the world's most universally used medicine. In addition to quieting pain, it also quiets joint inflammation and so is widely used by arthritics. Thus you can see that aspirin does double work for you if your back ailment is arthritis of the spine. One of the main drawbacks to aspirin is that it increases the acidity of the stomach. Therefore, if you have ever had a peptic ulcer, or have one now, aspirin is out. Instead your doctor may prescribe phenacetin or acetaminophen (under such trade names as Tylenol, Apamide, Nebs, and Tempra). Buffered aspirin (such as Ascriptin and Bufferin) or delayed dissolving aspirin may be allowed.

Other kinds of medicines that you may be given in the hospital are sedatives and tranquilizers. These are to slow you and your emotions and calm your anxieties.

Among the sedatives you may be given are barbiturates such as phenobarbital. This is to help calm you down and let you sleep for long periods. After all, you are in the hospital to rest, since rest is good for your back. Therefore, your doctor may feel that you need some medicine to help you rest and he may prescribe a barbiturate. Or, if he sees that you are worried and have not left your anxieties outside the hospital door, he may prescribe a tranquilizer pill such as Librium, Valium, Equanil, or Miltown.

In addition to relaxing your fears, some of these tranquilizers also chemically relax your muscles. In medical terms, they are muscle relaxants. There are also pills used primarily to relax muscles—such as your spastic back muscles —and incidentally work to also relax your emotions. Among the most widely used are Robaxin, Skelaxin and Sinaxar. Unfortunately, there is no medicine yet made, or even being experimented with, that can selectively relax the spastic muscles that cause backache—despite the claims in advertisements of the wonders of general muscle relaxants.

All of these medicines mentioned so far are taken as pills or are injected so as to get into your blood stream and act generally. There are, however, two kinds of injection treat-

ments that are specifically applied in the small of your back
right at the source of your problem. Since neither requires a
surgical operation, but are generally performed in the hospital, we'll describe them here.

In the case of arthritis of the spine, when the irritation can
be pinpointed to specific vertebral bones that are rubbing
against each other, a combination of painkiller and steroid
hormone may be injected. The painkiller is likely to be pro-
caine (Novocain) or one of the other "-caines." The steroid
hormone is a synthetic derivative of cortisone, the arthritis
wonder drug of the 1950's. The most usually used are hydro-
cortisone, prednisone and prednisolone. These are powerful
steroid hormones that can bring on other problems, such as
muscle weakness and peptic ulcer and can worsen existing
metabolic conditions, such as diabetes, so they are used carefully. They are seldom used on a daily or even weekly basis.
More likely, if you do receive such injections you'll receive
a couple during your hospitalization only, as a way to dra-
matically quiet the arthritic flare-up.

The other kind of injection, used only in cases of herniated
or ruptured disks, is still new and experimental as of this
writing (1971). It has been so successful in the 1,500 patients
on whom it has been tried around the world that its origina-
tor, Dr. Lyman Smith of Elgin, Illinois, advocated its wide
use and urged the U. S. Food and Drug Administration to ap-
prove it. Dr. Smith calls the injection procedure *chemonucle-
olysis*. It is based on the fact that an enzyme derived from the
papaya plant, called chymopapain, has the ability to dissolve
the material that has been squeezed out of a herniated disk.
Thus by chemically dissolving the extruded nucleus pulposus
(that's what chemonucleosis means), the enzyme melts away
the material that has been pressing on a nerve root and causing pain and spasm. You should know, although we'll talk
about it in a later chapter, that one of the most common surgi-

cal operations for slipped disk is the removal of just this material by knife. The primary advantage of the injection technique is that it makes the operation unnecessary in simple cases where squeezed-out disk material is the only problem.

If you have this injection, you'll be carted to the X-ray department and placed on a table of an X-ray machine, similar to one you may have been on during your diagnostic tests. This machine, however, is a fluoroscope. It projects the X-ray shadowgraph on a television screen so that the doctor can tell exactly what he is doing every split second. Before he inserts the needle, your back will be anesthetized so that you will feel no pain during the procedure. Some doctors go further, performing the procedure with their patients asleep under general anesthesia. They claim they do this because their patients are then less likely to move during the injection. So the enzyme injection may be done in an operating room.

In any case, a long needle is carefully positioned into the side of the space between two vertebrae—usually the space L5–S1. Then a little radiopaque substance is injected to be certain that the tip of the needle is near the disk protrusion. Next the enzyme solution is injected, and finally the needle is pulled out. The whole thing takes about 15 minutes. You're returned to your room and given painkillers and muscle relaxants. Ironically, the needle in your back may have set off a new muscle spasm and now this has to be treated until it subsides.

In the meantime, the enzyme acts specifically on the offending disk material. The enzyme does not affect surrounding bone, nerve roots, nerve casing, ligaments or blood vessels. But the protruding disk material melts away and diffuses through the other tissues of the body.

Studies of this enzyme injection on patients with herniated disks at Elgin, St. Louis, Texas, and elsewhere indicate that you can expect your sciatic pains to leave in about 24 hours.

You should be able to sit and walk on the second day and leave the hospital on the fifth to seventh day. Once home you can go back to work slowly, on a part-time basis at first. You should be back working full time in three to five weeks. That's about half the recovery time from a disk operation. And there are no stitches to be taken out!

No matter what kind of treatment you received in the hospital, you'll be gradually moved out of the bed. There's no trick to your back's feeling better in bed. The test of your progress is how it feels when you sit up and stand and hesitatingly take your first steps.

You'll be stiff at first. And you may feel a little lightheaded from having stayed in bed for so long. Just give your circulatory system a chance to readjust to your vertical position after having been horizontal. If you try to pop right out of bed after a week or so of rest, you may fall flat on your face as your blood drains and you faint. That's what happened to Ted after his hospitalized bed stay.

The usual procedure is for you to sit up at the edge of your bed at first, and let your legs dangle over the side. Then get up and go to the washroom when you need to. Then shower. Then walk around the room, and finally walk down the hall. At any point, if your back hurts, you'll be taken back to bed and you'll have to rest some more.

Finally, however, your back will no longer hurt. You'll be ready to go home. Before you leave, your doctor may construct a plaster cast over your trunk, to prevent you from bending your back and hurting it again. That's what the doctor did for Ted. Or he may order a corset, brace or back support made of cloth and reinforced with steel stays. These are also intended to keep your back from flexing and to help support it and help it to maintain its proper curvature. As it is fitted on you in the brace shop, you'll be given instructions on its use and how to keep it clean.

When you leave the hospital walking straight, you'll be a lot happier than when you arrived bent in pain and spasm. You'll be going home for the interim stage of your rest and treatment. You'll be leaving with instructions on how to live with your back at home in the next month or so—instructions that in a big way you'll have to follow for the rest of your life. We'll talk about these in the next chapter.

# 6. Treating Your Back at Home

Coming home from the hospital is always more pleasant than leaving home to go to the hospital. It's good to be home even if you've only been hospitalized for three days (chances are greater that you have been in the hospital longer, probably for ten days). When you left for the hospital, you were filled with anxieties and fears. This was only natural. Maybe, like Ted, you were doubly fearful because you visited your doctor in pain and on his advice suddenly went straight to the hospital from his office, without even packing an overnight bag.

As you return to your familiar home surroundings, you may breathe a sigh of relief, feeling that you can go back to the comfortable privacy of your personal life that contrasts so with the public openness that is hospital life. Only half of this feeling is correct, however. While your home is more comfortable and familiar and private than the hospital, you are not going back to all your old ways. You may slowly go back to *most* of your old ways, but certainly not to *all*. You have to somewhat alter your life activities at work and at play so that you can greatly increase the odds against having recurrence of your back trouble and of the terrible pain that came with it.

It may very well be that you are a reader who has not gone to the hospital. Your doctor may have told you to rest and to care for your back at home. If so, there is much useful information for you in the previous chapter on hospital care of your back. This chapter will also be useful to you, as well as for the back patient who has returned home from the hospital.

In either case, the theme of home care is to promote the healing of the disorder causing your pain and to extend the treatment your doctor prescribed.

You can't see the healing going on, as you can see healing progress in a cut on the skin. What's going on in your spine (or near it) is out of sight and thus rather mysterious. But you should realize that the process of healing is pretty much the same in all parts of the body. While it sounds trite, this ability of your body to heal is one of the miracles of life. Just remember that even in prehistoric times man's back troubles healed. They may have healed in crippling or even painful ways, but they did heal. However, the trick as we approach the twenty-first century is to promote the proper kind of healing that will return you to a normal and active life.

Muscles and ligaments usually can repair minor injuries by adding new cells to replace damaged ones and fill in tears in tissue. But the cells need to grow in a muscle that is behaving normally. If the muscle is in tight spasm, the muscle repair may be distorted. Nerves that have been injured can usually repair themselves by slowly generating new fibers.

Where there has been extensive damage, the body will "knit" scar tissue in the injured muscle or around the damaged nerve. In the case of tendons that have been injured, there is no other repair technique but scar tissue.

Scar tissue is elastic and tough. It tends to contract, like any elastic band. The benefit of exercise and posture control is to keep stretching the scar tissue so that it assumes a proper shape and size when it "sets."

Heat keeps your muscles relaxed and relieves spasms, dilates blood vessels to provide a rich blood supply to the healing area and generally works to enhance the entire healing environment. You are not likely to have diathermy or ultrasonic treatment machines at home since they are very expensive. The best kind of heat to apply at home is moist heat. There are three good ways to apply it. Each should be applied while you are supine, or lying on your back. Each should be tested to be pleasantly warm, not burning hot.

1. *Hot Pack*. This is simply a towel that has been soaked in hot water, then wrung out so that the heat remains as most of the water is squeezed away. Even so, it is a bit messy, especially if you are in bed. You might want to put a plastic sheet or rubber mat under you to keep from soaking your sheets and mattress. Obviously, the towels are going to cool, so your spouse, parent or friend is going to have to replace the cooled ones with fresh, warm ones periodically, probably every five minutes or so.

2. *Warm Bath*. A problem here is that you have to get in and out of the tub, and with a bad back that may not be too easy. It can be dangerous if you lose your foothold. It's best to hold tightly to hand grips as you get in and out; better yet, someone should be there to help you. Don't make the water too hot or you may invite other problems, such as raising your blood pressure. Always test the water before going in: someone flushing a toilet could have altered the water temperature you set when you first turned on the faucet. You don't want the water so hot it will burn. It's a good idea to have someone in earshot who can talk to you once in a while. Falling asleep in one's own bathtub can be very dangerous,

and more likely if you are on medication. Such accidents account for the fact that so many people can be drowned so far from a river, lake, or ocean: in the safety of their homes. Rest on your back in bed for half an hour to a full hour after you soak.

3. *Electric Heating Pad.* This is probably the most convenient way to apply heat to your back at home. Merely plug in the cord to a wall outlet, place the pad under your back, turn it on, and if it has an adjustment, set it to "low" or "medium" (never "high"). The pad is even more effective if you enclose it with a damp towel. But before you do so, be sure that it is the kind totally enveloped in plastic and guaranteed to be "wetproof." This should be stated on the label of the pad or on the box it comes in. If the pad comes with a cloth slipcase, look inside to see if the wetproof or waterproof guarantee is there. Most electric heating pads sold today are wetproof. But not all. And many people still have around their homes old flannel cloth heating pads. The point is that if the heating wires inside get wet, they might short-circuit and severely burn or even electrocute you. But if the pad is made of watertight plastic and all of the wiring is thus protected, you can safely enclose the pad in moist towels (the way we used to enclose hot-water bottles in towels). This, in effect, gives you warm packs that you don't have to renew every so often. Finally do not turn on the pad before you go to sleep for the night.

You'll probably do best with two heat treatments a day, each about 15 minutes long. You can vary the techniques and, for instance, use warm packs in the morning and a hot bath at night. In any case, you should only take one bath a day.

We can't emphasize enough how important heat treatments are for your back. In fact, in many subacute cases, it's better for you to stay home, lie down and apply heat to your back than to further insult your back by the walking, driving your car, riding a bus or taxi, climbing up and down stairs, dressing and undressing, it takes to leave your house and go to the hospital or doctor's office.

Many people feel that they can apply heat to their aching back by using liniment and ointments. You should know that they are dead wrong. Such popular self-treatments do no more than make your skin feel warm. The most widely used of such treatments contain turpentine, chloroform or wintergreen ointment. Muscle liniment is usually made of turpentine and chloroform. All of these are useless as far as bringing any heat to bear on your bad back. Their heat effect is only a skin sensation and does not penetrate the top layers of the skin. Wintergreen ointment does contain a small amount of methyl salicylate, an aspirin-like chemical, which may find its way to the bloodstream. But you would be better off taking two aspirins. In short, stay away from muscle liniment and ointments.

As when you were in the hospital, your doctor may want you to take certain medicines. Since he has allowed you to go home, you should not be in excruciating pain, requiring the very strong painkillers such as morphine and Demerol. Also you are likely now to be taking oral medicines, not the injected kind. Depending on how bad your pain still is, you may be taking codeine or aspirin. You are probably still taking a tranquilizer or muscle relaxant to calm your emotions and your back and trunk muscles. If you're having trouble sleeping, you may be still taking barbiturates, although this is less likely than in the hospital, since you are more active at home.

This applies to all of the medicine your doctor prescribes: follow the instructions on the label. If a little is good, a lot may be *not* better but worse. Also, if the instructions say "take three times a day," take the medicine at equal time intervals three times a day. A medicine should be administered so as to be constantly effective, keeping its level in the blood as constant as possible by taking it at evenly spaced intervals.

Another thing to consider when taking medicine is that the medicine—particularly a barbiturate—can make you feel "dopey" and thus uncertain about when you last took it. It is better, therefore, to let someone else give you the medicine.

Finally, be sure all your medicines are out of the reach of small children. And in this age of drug abuse, you should also keep the medicines out of reach of curious adolescents, too, as well as all other people who are looking for pharmacological kicks.

At home, as in the hospital, one of the chief treatments of your back condition is rest in bed. The reasons are the same: to allow your back to relax. It's that simple. Bed rest merely but profoundly relieves the back of its usual job of remaining vertical. This means that the spinal and trunk muscles, the associated ligaments and tendons, the intervertebral disks and the spinal joints don't have to work: therefore, they can rest.

Rest stops many of the causes of inflammation and spasm and promotes the proper healing processes. Make sure your mattress is firm and supportive and neither as rigid as a board nor as soft as a down pillow. (This is discussed in more detail in Chapter 9.)

As your mattress should properly support your spine when you are lying down, so your doctor may prescribe for you a *back support* to help you when you are sitting, standing and walking.

Back supports, also called *surgical corsets* or *braces,* are affectionately known by wearers as girdles. Usually they are not made of elastic, as are girdles, but of heavy cotton or nylon cloth, and surround most of the trunk. There are lots of so-called supports, sacral and otherwise, sold in drug stores and elsewhere, that claim to support the back. But your doctor knows that these are, like too many over-the-counter health products, designed less to help you, the patient, than the manufacturer and seller who make handsome profits from these essentially worthless products.

That's why your doctor will send you to a corsetmaker who specializes in the making of back supports and who takes customers only on doctors' recommendations. The corset that will be made for you will have these requirements: it will be snugly anchored to your pelvis (the anchor of your spine, remember) and extend up to the base of the breasts; it will have two light steel bars properly bent to the curve of your back, one immediately on each side of your spine. Some corsets have two additional steel bars a few inches farther from these, also parallel with the spine. All have a lacing or buckle arrangement in the front for tightening the corset so that it fits snugly.

You'll probably find the corset rather uncomfortable at first, especially around the chest, since it restricts movement and breathing. The whole idea of the corset is to limit the movements of your spine, allowing your spine to continue to curve properly no matter what you try to do while the corset is on. And as you sit or stand (which you'll be doing more of) your spinal and trunk muscles won't have to do all the work.

As you go into a back support for the first time, you are also starting a new phase of treatment. It's an interim phase, one between a past of total bed rest and a future phase of resumed activities. Wearing your back support, you can now sit up and read or talk and you can even walk around the house.

This is also true if your doctor starts you out in a plaster cast, as happened to Ted. You should have to wear the cast only for about a month. After that, you'll be fitted for a corset. Doctors who put their patients in body casts first do so to be absolutely sure that their patients don't get into trouble by flexing their spine or twisting it. You can't forget to put on a cast: it's a permanent fixture on you until it is sawed off. Incidentally, sawing off a cast these days is a cinch. Your doctor will use a special kind of vibrating saw that rips through the plaster in seconds, yet should it encounter flesh, it does not cut at all. It is based on the principle that your flesh will merely shake with certain vibrations but plaster will break with these same vibrations.

You shouldn't wear your back support all day. Wear it when you are up and around, but not while you are in bed. Also, keep it clean. The steel bars slip out of their special pockets so that you can launder the corset. After it is washed in mild suds and rinsed in cold water, it should be dried gently. If you use strong detergents and hot drying, the cloth will shrink and you'll be uncomfortable, or it will weaken and the seams will open.

If your back was strained, your doctor may have put layers of adhesive tape on it. This is to limit its motion so that you don't further injure it. The taping of backs is most often done for athletic injuries—especially in weekend athletes like Ted. He, remember, first hurt his back at golf, which is one of the most common causes of back strain. Beginners, particularly because of their lack of follow-through, have the most golf injuries. And practice strokes are the most dangerous because they often are jerky actions and because they occur in rapid succession (without any walking time in between).

Another new element of your care on the road to rehabilitation, is exercise. Chapter 10 describes exercises in detail. Right now we want to emphasize that you should start slowly and gently. The last thing you want to do now is sprain, strain or overexert. But you do want to limber up and you do need to start getting those trunk muscles back in shape. Remember, your muscles were probably much abused when you were put to bed. Then they rested and relaxed. Muscles that are not used, however, atrophy, or wither, and weak muscles can only cause you more back troubles. So the proper course now that you are feeling better and are at home is to start exercising those muscles to bring them up to shape, where they can properly support your spine. Then keep them in shape. Chapter 10 tells about that too.

Slowly, you'll be able to resume the full activities of your life again. In about a week you'll be walking around the block; in two weeks you'll be rarin' to go. It's good that you feel that way, but you should use some self-restraint, or else your family should restrain you. Don't start running the mile again. Don't go back to work on the freight dock right away. Don't go back to the office right away either. Instead, start resuming your former activities in stages. Go back to work for a couple of hours a day at first. Then increase this to half a day. If you feel fatigued, go home. After a couple of weeks of part-time work, and if you feel strong enough, then go back to work full-time—always remembering that you should take a rest period or even go home early when you feel tired, or if your back starts to ache.

It's too bad that more employers aren't enlightened enough to allow their back-injured workers (and others who have been in the hospital) to come back to work on a graded basis. Instead, they take the attitude that either you can work or you can't. That means either full-time or none at all: "If you can't work all day, then don't bother to come in." In these days of enlightenment about the medical needs of workers on the part of unions and management, you would think that at least the bigger industries would have graded back-to-work adjustments for employees getting back on their feet. We hope this will happen soon. End of sermon.

You should not go back to work even part-time unless your doctor agrees that you are fit for it. There is another consideration. You should not still be taking the kind of medication that produces effects that are safe enough at home, but that could be dangerous in some work situations. For instance, there is probably no harm done when a sedative makes you drowsy and you drop off to sleep in your easy chair. But if you get drowsy at work, and your job is driving a truck or operating a paper cutter, then you could have a serious accident. The other side to being medicated is this: if you are still taking heavy doses of a painkiller, you may still have a serious medical problem and may *not* be ready to return to work.

Back at work, you'll be feeling stronger every day and you will be attempting to do more every day. That's fine, providing you do things right. That means sitting properly and standing properly, and no lifting—if these are involved in your job. All this is covered later, in Chapter 9, which you should reread until you know it by heart.

With your renewed strength will come a renewed interest in sports. But before you attempt even the mildest of athletic activities, be sure that your muscles are back in shape. Specific exercises to return them to shape are detailed in Chapter 9, as well as a thorough run-down on which calisthenics and athletic activities are good, and which bad, for your back.

If you're feeling better, you're probably wondering about your sexual activity too. Don't wonder. We'll be quite explicit, because sex is an important part of most adults' lives.

Sex was probably the furthest thing from your mind when you had your backache attack. But now that you are recuperating, the idea and the feeling should be returning. That's good. It is a sign that you are recovering physically and emotionally from your acute back attack.

Before you took to bed with your back, you probably made love when you and your partner felt like it, and in any way that pleased you. Much of this still applies, but with a few cautions that should merely limit your positions, not your participation and enjoyment.

After what we've said about returning to activities, the first precaution is probably obvious: take it easy. Resume your activities on a gradual build-up basis. Don't rush right into exotic postures and positions immediately.

On the other hand, your sexual ingenuity will be freshly challenged now. Ted, for instance, remembers that when he returned from the hospital he had a chest-to-pelvis plaster cast and yet was able to devise ways of having mutually satisfying sexual intercourse with his wife, even though she was in an advanced stage of pregnancy at the time!

To be very explicit, there are two important principles to keep in mind. One is that the erect penis is at an angle of 25 degrees, so any position of the man's partner that allows the vagina to meet this angle will be satisfying and provide the proper friction that results in climax. The other principle is that the partner with the bad back should flex that back (bend it forward) as little as possible, or not at all. Now, in the most common position of sexual intercourse, the so-called missionary position, the woman is supine and the man is above, face to face. To slide his penis in and out of her vagina requires movement of the small of the back just at the usual trouble spot of L4 and L5 disks. This reciprocating action alternates the position of the spine from humpback (or flexion) on insertion to swayback on withdrawal. Thus, the man on top with a bad back can pop a disk or unstable vertebra when he pulls back, or can painfully stretch his sciatic nerve when he moves forward.

The way to avoid this is for the person with the bad back to be on the bottom, with his back against the mattress, letting the partner do the humping. The man or woman on the bottom is in the gatched position, which is good for the spine.

Some men are hung up on being "the one on top" and see it as a symbol of dominating their female partner. Rubbish! Now is the time to give your sex life a little variety, a chance to leave the staid and usual and be saucy and try some new positions. Try it lying on your sides, either in face-to-face or rear-entry positions—with the partner with the good back doing the humping motions.

Don't let your bad back keep you from sex or other activities. Don't use it as an excuse for not taking part in the pleasures of life. Too many men, particularly, regard their bad backs as a sign of weakness, of some erosion of their masculinity. This sad but real fact of life was highlighted in a 1966 study of 43 men with bad backs who were seen at Ohio State University Hospital.[1] The doctors who made the study realized that certain nerves could be damaged and thus remove the ability of a patient to have an erection, particularly the nerves with roots at L2, L3 and L4. But in studying cases reported by other doctors they found such nerve damage was rare. "For every case of organic impotence reported there are at least nine cases of psychologic impotence," they discovered. In talking to the 43 Ohio patients whose backs had been injured on the job, the doctors found that 16 were able to have erections and sexual intercourse, but that 27 of the men could not—by definition, they were impotent. Furthermore, their impotence stemmed back to the time of their back injury, but was not physically caused by it. The researchers found that the reasons for the men's impotence varied, but were all purely psychological. Mostly, these were men who had been the "babies" of their family (the youngest or only child). Now that their backs were somewhat disabled, the men reverted to their babied ways; some even let their wives go to work and become the breadwinners and head of the house, while they stayed home and became increasingly passive.

Many of these men returned to their masculine roles as husband and father after rehabilitation in the Ohio hospital. The men had to learn that they were not "back cripples."

Our point should be rather obvious now. Whether you are

[1]Myron M. LaBan, Richard D. Burk, and Ernest W. Johnson, "Sexual Impotence in Men Having Low-Back Syndrome," *Archives of Physical Medicine* (November 1966), *47*:715-723.

a man or a woman with a bad back, don't let it cripple you psychologically or physically. A back cripple is a sad thing to see: a person afraid to do things. Don't be afraid to do anything providing you do it in a way that maintains the proper curve of your spine. If you lie around and do nothing, your muscles and your emotional health will wither from disuse. Either of these atrophies, or both, can cause a worsening of your back condition.

If you find that even though you really try, you cannot get up and around, talk to your doctor. It may well be that you need the advice of another kind of professional, such as a social worker or even a psychiatrist. There is no shame in going for such help; that's what they are there for. And they are as much health professionals as your family physician or orthopedist.

While you are home, you should be careful about your diet. In the hospital this is taken care of for you, but at home you and whoever prepares your meals have to plan ahead. Your diet should be nutritious, with sufficient proteins, carbohydrates, fats and minerals to keep you healthy enough to repair your back trouble, but not so caloric that you gain weight from your limited activity. If you have gout, watch the purines; if you have diabetes, watch the sugar. Also, be sure you get enough vitamins, even if you have to take a vitamin pill every day.

You should also schedule your time wisely, so that as you resume activities you still have periods of rest. Maintain fairly regular hours, eat meals regularly and give yourself enough sleep every night. Remember, you've got healing to do, so you have to provide your body with as much opportunity to heal as possible.

Your doctor will probably want to see you only once a month for the two or three months after you start to care for your back at home. But that doesn't mean you shouldn't call him between visits if you feel something isn't right.

If you have any questions about what activities you should try, call him before trying them.

If you feel any pain or spasm of your back, call him.

If you start to experience any unusual symptoms, call him. These might well be side reactions caused by the medication you are taking. If you are having bad reactions from one medicine, he can put you on another that can relax your muscles, or whatever, without producing unwanted reactions. You can save both of you a lot of trouble if you tell him in advance about reactions these drugs may have caused you in past illnesses. Also, before you take any medicine, you should tell your doctor if you have any of these other conditions:

    drug addiction
    epilepsy
    glaucoma or other eye disorder
    heart trouble
    peptic ulcer
    diabetes
    asthma, emphysema or other breathing disorder
    kidney trouble (including stones)
    liver disease

Among the adverse reactions you should watch for and tell your doctor about are:

    heartburn
    nausea
    vomiting
    constipation
    diarrhea
    stomachache
    blood in stools or vomit
    dizziness
    ringing in the ears
    headache
    fatigue

skin rash
confusion
lack of physical coordination
drowsiness and lethargy
irritability
blurred vision
fast or slow heartbeat
breathing difficulties

You can see that for the most part your recovery at home is in your own hands and in the hands of your family. If everyone cooperates, your back will heal and you'll be a new person. By all means be optimistic. You ARE getting better and you will soon be able to do just about everything—and enjoy it.

Since you are better, you have avoided the need for an operation, which is the subject of the next two chapters. So skip them and go on to Chapter 9, where you will learn about the new ways you'll be doing things. The new and SAFE ways.

# 7. Your Back Operation

When you talk to friends who have back problems, you're liable to find one who proudly tells you that he hasn't had any troubles since his back was operated on. And he will try to sell you on the idea of having your own operation, asking what kind of doctor you have, how long your back has been hurting and so forth.

There is no more zealous missionary about any treatment than a patient for whom the treatment has worked. He relates his experience just as fervently as a religious convert or someone who has just given up smoking.

Alas, nothing in life is that simple. Surgery may turn out to be the final and best answer to your back problem. And being the most dramatic, it makes for good conversation with beer or cocktails. But it is the most drastic of treatments. And as safe as modern surgical techniques and modern anesthesia are, they are still not without their dangers. No therapy is. That's why your doctor will try out every other appropriate form of treatment for your back before he advises surgery.

It may be that you have gone the route of ten days in the

hospital, ten days at home, and your back is still killing you. Or the pain is still there in your leg. Or your toe is still as numb as ever. Or the injection of cortisone into the space between vertebrae only temporarily quieted your arthritis. You've worn a back support and done your exercises and limited your physical work—and you are still in agony. After about six weeks of such intensive but nonsurgical treatment your doctor may suggest that you have surgery.

Of course, he will weigh other factors besides the considerable one of your misery. He realizes that there is no magic in any treatment, even in today's miraculous surgery. After all, any operation is a heavy dose of stress on the body. One big question is: Is the condition worth the stress? There's another question: Can your body take the stress?

You should be pleased, rather than impatient with your doctor's conservatism. After all, it's your health and life that are at stake. Your doctor, if he is wise, knows that the best healer on earth is nature. He will try to best help nature heal. If rest, heat and support fail, only then might he consider surgery for you. Once he has decided that an operation is what you need, he will help bring all of modern surgical skill to bear on your back problem.

Of course, the opposite might be the case. It may be that he has recommended surgery on your back and *you* have been delaying. Perhaps other people have been telling you how horrible surgery is. Or perhaps you remember the days when your tonsils were removed or your nose prettied.

Remember, though, that your doctor is recommending it. He is your doctor because you have faith in his skills and knowledge. Therefore, you ought to take his advice. And you can rest assured that if the surgery is performed in an accredited hospital it has to be good. Surgeons do not operate in isolation, accountable to no one, as they did a century ago. Today there are eyes on him in the operating room. Furthermore, every bit of tissue that is removed from every patient in a hospital is microscopically examined by his critical fellow doctors. This is the Tissue Committee. Every hospital has one today. If it finds that tissue was removed from a patient for no good reason, the surgeon who removed it stands to lose all his operating room privileges unless he can otherwise prove it was necessary.

There are situations in which the nature of your back trouble qualifies for an operation, but *you* don't. You may have a disease, such as uncontrolled diabetes or hemophilia (bleeder's disease) or severe emphysema, which would provide more of a threat than could be justified in an operation. Or perhaps you're suffering from malnutrition, or you are grossly overweight, or you are going through an emotional crisis.

Your doctor has to weigh all these factors when he considers surgery as the best treatment for your back now.

You can probably tell from reading this book thus far which back conditions are likely candidates for surgery. Such acute conditions as fractured vertebrae (broken back) and massive rupture of a disk are often taken into the operating room on an emergency basis. Sciatica and spondylolisthesis are frequent reasons for prompt spinal surgery. Infections, tumors and arthritis are less frequent but still urgent reasons for surgery.

There are essentially two kinds of back operations. One is to relieve pressure on nerves by removing the material causing the pressure, usually material from a herniated disk. The other is to stabilize the back, to lock adjoining vertebrae together so that there is no motion between them. Both kinds of operations are usually done under general anesthesia, but often under local anesthesia. They are performed while you are prone, lying face down, on the operating table.

Since the pressure-relieving operations are simpler, let's take them first. In Chapter 5 we told about the procedure in which a needle is inserted between vertebrae and an enzyme injected that dissolves the disk material impinging on a nerve. We mention it here because in some hospitals this is performed in the X-ray department, but in other hospitals it is performed in the operating room, even though no incision is made. (For more details, see pages 66-68.)

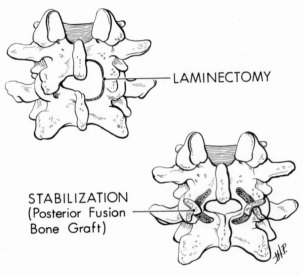

LAMINECTOMY

STABILIZATION
(Posterior Fusion
Bone Graft)

*Back operations. The two most common kinds of operations for back trouble are the laminectomy and the stabilization. In the first the lamina is chiseled open, and loosened bits of disk are cut away. In the second, bone is grafted to prevent vertebrae from moving (shown here is the Hibbs operation).*
*Fig. 5*

The surgical procedure for removing this impinging disk material is often called a *laminectomy*, so-named because the lamina—that thin plate of bone that forms the back oblique angles of the spinal canal—is removed in order to get at the offending disk material. Actually the laminectomy proper is midway in the entire operation. The operation begins with an incision about four inches long made just in the middle of the spine over the troublesome vertebrae. The incision is made through the skin and through the posterior ligament that runs down the back of the spine. Then this flesh is pulled aside, or retracted, exposing the bony vertebrae itself. The surgeon will carefully chisel or saw an opening in this bone (to one side or the other of the spinous process) about the size of a penny or nickel. He has to be very careful to not involve the facets on either side—unless he intends to also fuse them, as we'll explain later.

Using a bright surgical spotlight, he looks into the tunnel he has made through skin, muscle, ligament and bone and very carefully notes the material pressing on the spinal nerves. The myelogram taken a day or two before may be right in the operating room to accurately guide the surgeon in his next moves. With extreme gentleness, he moves the spinal nerves aside. At last the offender is isolated, ready to be removed. In most cases it is the white pea-sized disk matter that has popped out from between the vertebrae. The disk was pretty well degenerated when that happened, so that it is no longer its bouncy gelatinous self, but is now a fibrous stringy material that surgeons say is much like crabmeat. With a long instrument, the surgeon snips out strands of this "crabmeat" that have imposed pressures on the nerve roots and takes it away. This is *excision*, another term for this procedure.

At best, the surgeon can excise about half of the diseased disk. He cannot go all of the way through the diameter of the vertebral space because there is terrible danger ahead: if he pierces the thin anterior ligament that runs in front of the spine he may nick the aorta, which runs alongside it. Any damage to the aorta, which is the thickest artery in the body and which carries fresh blood from the heart, can result in hemorrhage. The death of a movie actor was attributed to just such an occurrence in 1961. Fortunately, such occurrences are very rare; unfortunately this means that there is still "crabmeat" between the vertebrae that may break loose and impinge on a nerve root at some time in the future, although this is not likely.

Sometimes the material pressing on a nerve root is not squeezed from a disk. Sometimes it is made of fragments of bone that were broken during a fracture of the vertebrae. Sometimes it is made of bony spurs or deposits from arthritis. It can also be used to relieve pressures of infections. Rarely is it a tumor. In all of these conditions, too, the operation may involve opening the laminae of more than one vertebrae—chiseling openings in more than one backbone.

A laminectomy–excision operation takes about an hour and a half.

The other kind of back operation is designed to stabilize or stop motion between adjoining vertebrae. Technically it is *arthrodesis,* but commonly it is called a *fusion* operation because it involves the fusion, or biological gluing of bone into a solid mass. Fusion is always the technique used to treat slipped vertebrae, or spondylolisthesis. It is also used to treat broken vertebrae and vertebrae that have been attacked by tuberculosis or arthritis. Spinal fusion is also done by many surgeons in combination with excision for slipped disk.

Usually two neighboring vertebrae are fused (L4 and L5 and L5 and S1 are the most common combinations) to keep them from moving.

The fusion operation, when performed alone and not in combination with others, begins with an incision in the skin down the middle of the spine. Then the muscles and the posterior ligament (which runs down the back of the spine) are cut and retracted. After this, any of several procedures may be followed. All contain the same elements: the bone along the back at selected sites is cut with a chisel and mallet, layer by layer, until bleeding bone is reached. Then equally raw bone is taken from another part of the body and wedged, wired or fastened with ivory screws to the vertebrae. This is actually a bone graft, or bone transplant.

You should understand that bone grafts work differently than do grafts of soft tissue, such as corneal grafts used in the eye or even whole-heart transplants. Once bone is sawed or chiseled away from its blood supply it starts to die. But when it is placed tightly against raw living bone, it serves as a trellis upon which new bone can grow from the living bone.

You may, like many people, think of bone as solid ivory. Actually while bone looks rather solid when you see it in museum skeletons, it is in fact hollow. Bone is hard and tough, but it contains many hollow channels of blood vessels. And at the core of bone is yellow marrow, a substance rich in blood supply that manufactures red blood cells.

Here are some of the things that go on in a bone graft. First a blood clot forms on the open bone wound. Then tiny channels are formed that conduct *fibroblasts* (the repair cells of the body), which sort of cement the bone pieces together. The bond is a form of cartilage, which attracts *osteoblasts,* the bone-forming cells of the body. These cells construct osteoid tissue, a protein framework on which is deposited mineral calcium, to complete the bonemaking. At the same time as bone is being made, another kind of cell, *osteoclasts*, take the old bone trellis and cartilage tissue away, bit by bit. The entire process takes about four months (compared to the six weeks it takes a fracture to heal).

The bits of bone that are grafted to your back bone in a fusion operation may come from one of two sources—called *donor sites* by surgeons. One is the *iliac crest,* that ridge of bone you can feel under your beltline, which is the top of the pelvis. Some surgeons prefer to slice off some bone from the ilium because it is "succulent"—a medical term meaning it has a rich blood supply. This enhances its chances of "taking," while the cut ilium is better able to repair itself. Also, the surgeon can get some of that bone in the same operation, by making a hockey-stick-shaped incision that turns the corner from the spine to the iliac crest on the right or the left.

The slices of bone for your spinal fusion may be taken, instead, from your shin bone, or *tibia.* Some surgeons prefer tibia bone because it is stronger than the iliac bone, and patients say it hurts less during recovery, although it takes a second incision to remove.

There are many different ways to graft bone to vertebrae in order to "freeze" them. One of the most frequently used is called *Hibb's operation,* in which the vertebral bone is sort of knit together. It's done this way: the surgeon uses a steel instrument to peel back the top layer or *periosteum* on each side of the spinous process; he makes one slice up and one slice down. Then he joins the raw surfaces of these "bone peels" of neighboring vertebrae. Finally, he may fracture the spinous process and connect it to the vertebra below. Sometimes in this operation slices of bone from the hip or shin are grafted to join the edges of the vertebral bodies.

Another frequently used technique is the *H-graft,* also known as the *clothespin graft.* For this, a rectangular slice of bone is taken from the iliac or shin and notches are carefully cut at each end. Then the graft is fit so that the spinous process of one vertebra above and the one below wedge into the notches. The tips of the spinous processes, of course, were previously stripped to bleeding bone to assure that the graft would take. Often, small slices of bone are packed between the H-graft and the lamina, and other bone slices are inserted between the facets or intervertebral joints (previously stripped of their slippery cartilage faces). This may all be done while your spine is bent forward in flexion, so that the graft can immediately take weight and relieve pain.

Sometimes, for spondylolisthesis, surgeons perform what

they call the *Gill procedure,* otherwise known as the "un-roofing." This is the complete removal of the posterior elements of a vertebra: the laminae and spinous process. This is to remove the broad area of pressure on the nerve roots lying underneath. Then the unroofed vertebra is fused to vertebra above and below—usually with rectangles of transplanted bone grafted to the transverse processes at each side.

Many surgeons combine the excision and fusion operations for herniated disk, although the combination is still in dispute. The reason they combine them, they say, is "to stabilize the spine." This means that they want to keep the interval between vertebrae and preserve the space left behind by the removal of disk material. They hope to remove or reduce pressure on the remaining half of disk left between the vertebrae. They perform the fusion to give the ligaments and facets additional support.

Often, a surgeon doesn't know until he is operating and can see first-hand what is going on in your back, whether he'll do a single or combination operation. Certainly the combination excision–fusion operation is not for every bad back, or even for every slipped disk patient. Certainly, the combination operation takes longer (about three hours) and has a longer recovery and recuperation period.

At Mayo Clinic the combination excision–fusion operation has been on the increase since it was first used in 1938. In 1971, about half of all slipped disk patients received the combination surgery.[1] Meanwhile at Massachusetts General Hospital, in Boston, the combination has decreased in use.[2]

It's really too much for a patient like yourself to judge.

[1]Richard N. Stauffer, John C. Ivins, and Ross H. Miller, "The Lumbar Disc Syndrome and Its Operative Treatment," *Postgraduate Medicine,* (February 1971): 87-93.

[2]Joseph S. Barr et al., "Evaluation of End Results in Treatment of Ruptured Lumbar Intervertebral Disks with Protrusion of Nucleus Pulposus," *Surg. Gynec. Obstet.,* (1967): *125*:250-256.

Especially when the experts can't agree. Put yourself instead in the hands of an able surgeon with a good reputation that is backed by a high success rate and you can't go wrong.

You should know that there are two kinds of surgical specialists who operate on the spine. One is the *neurosurgeon*. The spine is his realm since it contains the spinal cord, which is, after all, the body's main bundle of nerves connecting to the brain. The other kind is an *orthopedic surgeon*. Sometimes you have a choice, sometimes the choice is made for you. For instance, there are orthopedic surgeons who won't operate on the spine. Most neurosurgeons will remove the material from a herniated disk that presses on a nerve root in the spine, but will not do spinal fusions. Sometimes the hospital will direct specialists to do one thing or the other. And sometimes both a neurosurgeon and an orthopedic surgeon may cooperate on your back operation. If they do, don't worry about getting a double bill. You will receive a bill from each specialist, but it will be for his *half* of the total job. Since one of the authors of this book (RGA) is an orthopedic surgeon, we are naturally partial to that kind of specialist for back operations. If you do pick an orthopedic surgeon (or orthopedist or orthopod), make sure he or she is one of the 4,474 (as of February, 1970) active Fellows of the American Academy of Orthopedic Surgery, which insures his professional stature and skills as being the highest.

Here's how to figure what your back operation may cost, at least a ball-park figure, as executives say.

*The Hospital:*

Your semiprivate room will cost about $85 a day (one to two weeks for laminectomy, two to three for fusion). The myelogram will cost about $40, and other X-rays probably another $45. You'll have to also pay for the operating room and the administration of anesthesia ($100 to $250). These costs should be covered by Blue Shield-Blue Cross or any other good medical-hospitalization insurance.

### *The Doctor:*

For a laminectomy–excision, the surgeon might charge $500 to $700. For an excision-and-fusion, his fee might be $600 to $900. Some or all of his fee should be covered by Blue Shield or any other good medical insurance.

# 8. Before and After Your Operation

Your back operation involves still more than we've yet told you. The previous chapter gave you the essential facts about the kinds of operations and when they are used because we felt that is what you wanted to know first. But you should also understand some facts about your *pre*operative and *post*-operative care.

Before your operation you will be thoroughly examined by the surgeon, even though your own family physician may have already carefully examined you. The surgeon will go over your X-rays and laboratory test results so that he knows everything about you that he can. He will also order tests to evaluate the state of health of your heart and lungs, your kidneys, the condition of your blood, and will search for hidden conditions such as diabetes, allergies and reactions to drugs that may require special consideration in surgery or that may (if severe enough) make surgery too dangerous.

The surgeon does not operate just because you walked into his office or because your physician referred you to him. He operates because he has made up his mind and is satisfied that surgery is your best option. Dr. A. V. Partipilo, clinical professor of surgery at Stritch School of Medicine, Loyola University, Chicago, put it well in his textbook, *Surgical Technique*: "The decision to operate should be based upon a careful consideration of the history, and a careful analysis of the physical and laboratory findings of each individual case, for each case presents a different and distinct problem."

When you go to the hospital for your operation, be sure to bring with you only the essentials:

No more than $5 in cash to pay for magazines, newspapers, etc., for the time you will feel well enough to thumb through them.

Travel clock.

Small radio.

Personal-sized TV (if allowed).

Toiletries such as toothbrush, toothpaste, comb, brush, shaving or cosmetic items.

Pajamas (two pairs), robe and slippers.

Nothing of value. Hospitals are public places, where such things often get lost or stolen.

In some hospitals, you fill out preadmission forms at home, then mail them in. If not, bring your Blue Cross-Blue Shield card or other identification of your hospitalization-major medical insurance plans, or else bring a checkbook to pay the hospital for its care. As we explained at the end of the previous chapter, back operations are expensive. But you have to remember that the hospital (unless it is one of the few remaining *proprietary* hospitals which are usually smaller) is a nonprofit community hospital. It therefore cannot and does not make any money. In fact, it loses money and that's why it has to ask for public donations every year to keep operating.

You will probably be admitted a day or two before your operation is scheduled to be performed. One reason for this is to allow time for X-rays and other tests. Another is to give the hospital team time to get you ready for the operation. For unless your surgery needs to be performed under emergency conditions, you will receive special care to prepare you. This will include fasting for 8 to 12 hours before the operation— since most surgery in hospitals is performed in the morning, this means your last food and drink will probably be your late-evening snack. The reason is to assure that your stomach is empty when you are being operated on. Otherwise, under anesthesia, it is possible for you to vomit and then choke on what you regurgitate, or cough or even suffocate. For a similar reason, you may also be given an enema before you go to sleep. Often the normal nervous strain of the occasion loosens bowels; this could be a disaster during the operation, not so much because of the offense to aesthetics but rather to the germ-free, aseptic conditions under which the operation must take place. You may also be given a sleeping pill the night before to assure adequate rest; chances are you're more than just a bit worried about undergoing surgery. Again, that's quite natural.

During the day or two before your operation, your surgeon will have spent much time getting—in his terms—your electrolytes in balance, meaning the state of minerals and nutrition of your bodily fluids. This is usually accomplished with diet, but sometimes intravenous fluids need to be given.

The night before, too, your back will be "prepped" by shampooing and shaving. Don't be surprised if the nurse shaves you from the shoulder blades down to the middle of your thighs. The purpose is to cleanse the area and to remove all the hair, which might otherwise harbor bacteria that could start an infection in your wound (the site of the surgery).

An hour or so before your operation you may be given a

powerful painkiller such as morphine or Demerol; a medicine for calming you down, such as Phenergan (promethazine) or Vistaril (hydroxuzine); and a medicine such as atropine or scopolamine to reduce bodily secretions.

Just before you are to be taken from your room you will have to empty your bladder. If you have a history of urinary retention, because of prostate enlargement, bladder infection or some other reason, a plastic or rubber tubing (catheter) will be inserted into your urethra. The other end of the tubing empties into a plastic bag, which will follow you into the operating room and back again to your room after the operation.

As you are lifted from your bed and placed on the cart, you may be alert enough to realize that you are feeling fine. Your euphoria is probably due to the medicine just injected into you. You may be so "high" that you can't understand why, as the ceiling lights in the corridor flash by, you feel so nice when, after all, you are about to be operated on. You will probably feel drowsy and may even doze off. There is a good chance you will not even remember being wheeled into the operating room. You may not be aware of anything again until you awaken after the operation in the recovery room and the nurse bending over you calls your name.

The anesthesiologist, a physician you may never see (or the anesthetist, who is a specially trained nurse) has selected with care the tranquilizers, sleep-inducers, and painkillers to use on you. He or she will insert into a vein in your hand or arm, foot or leg, a needle that will remain throughout your operation and for some hours thereafter. It is a pipeline into your body. Through it, at first, will be inserted some Pentothal (thiopental), which will put you to sleep. This is the beginning of your anesthesia. The anesthesiologist will wrap a pressure cuff around your upper arm so that he can continually measure your blood pressure—of vital importance during surgery.

Once you are asleep, the anesthesiologist will insert a plastic breathing tube into your mouth and throat (called an *endotracheal tube*). This is to give him control over your breathing and keep your airway constantly open. Through the tube he will let flow some halothane and nitrous oxide mixture or other anesthetic gases. (Local anesthesia, with an injection in the back, is sometimes used but not preferred.)

Then you will be lifted and gently turned over and placed on the operating table, face down. Remember you are now a dead weight, so it takes four or more people to lift you and turn you. You will be placed in what surgeons call the spinal rest position, with enough room for your chest to expand as you breathe and with your arms outstretched so that intravenous fluids can keep flowing into you.

A metal plate will be slipped under your thighs; it serves as "ground" for the electric cautery instrument that the surgeon will use to stop small "bleeders." Then the skin in a wide area around the troublesome vertebrae will be thoroughly scrubbed with soap and water and coated with a non-stinging iodine solution; this is to clear the area of all germs that might cause infection once the skin is cut open. Finally, your back will be covered with clean, sterile sheets so as to leave exposed only the area to be operated on.

With his team of scrub nurse, rotating nurse, assistant (always a doctor), anesthesiologist and perhaps a surgical student all ready, your surgeon will pick up a scalpel in his gloved, sterile hand and make the first incision.

After your surgery you will "come to" and regain consciousness either in the recovery room, or intensive care unit. Each is a special room with oxygen, many kinds of instruments and lots of nurses to care for your special post-operative needs. You'll be here for several hours as nurses watch you and help you to emerge from the anesthesia. They'll call your name and squeeze your hand, making sure that you respond and try to wake up. This is for your own good. You won't hurt but your natural reflexes will return with consciousness. If you have not urinated in eight hours, they will pass a catheter into your bladder to relieve it.

This is the worst time for your family. They may have been waiting for hours, thinking you were under the knife all this time. Actually, much of your big day has been spent waiting to get into the operating room for your surgery and then after the surgery, waiting in this special staging area where you can be closely watched until you are awake enough to be returned to your room. Most hospitals have a notification system for letting waiting friends and relatives know what is happening to you.

Back in your room and partially aware of your surroundings again, you'll notice that you are very thirsty. This is partly because of fluids lost in surgery and partly because the anesthetic gases are extremely dry. You may not have any appetite though. Don't worry; that's normal. So is a little nausea.

Your first two or three days will be painful ones. But the pain should be somewhat relieved by pills. However, if the pain becomes unbearable, don't suffer in silence. Let the nurse know. Or let your surgeon know when he visits you.

The trend in hospitals today is to get patients vertical as soon after surgery as possible. If you've had a disk removed (laminectomy or excision), you should be able to sit up in a day or two after surgery. Your nurse will help you up and persuade you to dangle your feet over the side of the bed. You'll be woozy at first, but that's because you've been horizontal for so long that your circulatory system has to slowly adjust to your being upright again. Your doctor wants you to start getting up and around because activity helps prevent pneumonia and also helps you to regain your strength faster than if you lie in bed constantly. It also helps to prevent the formation of blood clots in your veins.

On the other hand, don't try to do too much right away. How well you recover depends a great deal on how well you follow your surgeon's instructions during this crucial recuperation period. You'll be sitting in a chair, then taking your first steps in another day or two. If he soon has you walking to the toilet (fourth to sixth day), don't abuse the privilege by strolling down the corridor. He'll tell you when you may do that.

You will feel some discomfort in your back and you will be weak, and you may wonder how this is better than the acute attack that prompted the operation. Just remember that you'll soon recover from the surgery; you most likely would have had recurrent back attacks without it.

Don't worry about not moving your bowels. You won't be "regular" for a few weeks because of the shock this has imposed on your system. Interestingly enough, you may find that your bowels start behaving again just after your appetite comes back. And, after all, that's the way it should be!

As you can imagine, you're going to lose some weight during this period. That stands to reason since your food intake will be diminished for a while. But after a few weeks your weight should stabilize. That means you could easily put on pounds again. If you want to, that's fine. Otherwise watch your calories! If you needed the weight loss because you were overweight before, you can stay at your new lower weight, provided your doctor feels it is all right to do so. Remember, though, you need adequate nutrition to recover from the stress surgery has imposed and to heal properly.

If you've had the fusion operation, your surgeon will be less likely to want you moving around as early as he allows patients who have had only their disks cut. Remember that in *your* spine there are pieces of raw bone held or wedged together. To fuse, or solidify, they must stay firmly against each other. Any movement between them will interfere with or ruin the "take." So your doctor will want you on your back in bed for about a week after the operation. Then you'll start walking.

Also, you will have two places that hurt: the wounds over your spine and the donor site—that place where some bone was sliced away, either hip or shin.

A week or two later, before you are to be discharged from the hospital, you may have an X-ray taken of your back, just so the surgeon can evaluate how well the graft is placed. Also, before you leave you may be taken to the brace shop where a back support will be tailored for you. This is to limit the motion of your spine, especially of those vertebrae that are fusing. You'll probably have to wear the brace for months.

At home after the laminectomy, you'll be gaining strength every day. Stairs are a special problem and you should not try to climb any during the couple of weeks you'll be confined to the house. During your enforced stay at home, you should be doing more and more by stages: taking little walks around the block and sitting up longer and longer. If your job or occupation is sedentary—working in an office—you can most likely go back to work four to six weeks after surgery. If yours is work that includes heavy physical labor, you'd best wait for six to twelve weeks to get back on the job. That's quite a range, but it really depends on how well you are mending. Some doctors prescribe back supports for their patients returning to work.

After your fusion operation, you'll be sent home to stay for two or three weeks. Your activities will be much more restricted than those of laminectomy-only colleagues. If your occupation is of the sedentary kind, your doctor may let you go back to work on a limited basis in six to eight weeks. If your kind of work is physical, he'll keep you from it for six months. You can expect to wear your back support for anywhere from four to eight months after you leave the hospital.

What about sex after surgery? You won't be thinking about it for a long time, but when you start feeling better you certainly will. This is quite a healthy feeling. You can start resuming your sexual activities with your mate about one to two months after a disk operation and about three to six months after a fusion operation. If you haven't already read the section on sex in Chapter 6, you should. It gives good pointers about getting back in the erotic swing again, while still protecting your spine.

By now you've derived an idea of how serious a procedure surgery is. Now that you know what the operations are all about, and their recovery periods, the big question in your mind must be: Is it worth it all?

Only you can evaluate that as a yes or no answer. But let's look at what you might expect. After a laminectomy-excision operation, you'll probably find that the worst symptoms you had before the operation—numbness in the feet and especially the toes—are gone. The pain down your leg may be gone, but don't be too surprised if some residual pain takes time to disappear. Remember that those nerves were terribly irritated for a long time. For the same reason, there may be some residual numbness; it will take time for feeling to return; in some people, it never does.

After a fusion operation, there is also pain for a long time at the donor site. But all the pain should gradually fade.

You may wonder what fills up the hole after the offending disk material was cut away, after a small circle of laminal bone is chiseled out and after some bone was sliced away for a graft. The answer is: nothing. It's the same as when a diseased appendix or gall bladder is removed. The body tissue and its fluids, and some scar tissue, simply move into the small remaining space. And that is all.

As for your scars: they'll serve as small, visible trophies of your surgical experience only temporarily. Surgeons today know how to make very thin scars and after the stitches (sutures) are removed there will be little to see. And besides, scars pigment and blend in with your skin tone as time goes on. The scar itself is likely to be located at or below the belt line, so it is usually covered. It may itch, though, for a long time. In a real sense, that is nature's way of telling you that healing is going on there. After some months, you won't notice that anymore.

You should be very much aware of the problems and complications that are possible after back surgery. Wound infections and abscesses are always possible, but with today's germ-free techniques and antibiotics these rarely occur.

One of the most serious possible complications is pain. If you let your back condition deteriorate for too long, or if it deteriorated faster than you or your doctor realized, it is possible that some permanent damage was done to nerve roots in your spinal column. Such damage is rarely, maybe never, repaired satisfactorily by the body. The result could be pain you'll have to learn to live with, or some residual numbness that will also never go away. You also have to face the fact that your emotions can also cause backache.

There is always the possibility—and you must face it— that the operation will produce successful results for a while, perhaps years, and then your back will ache again. One reason may be that the disease process is just impossible to stop. Arthritis, for instance. Or the deep-seated remainder of the disk (which, remember, the surgeon couldn't cut out because it was too dangerously close to the aorta on the other side of the anterior ligament) could start shedding "crabmeat" pieces that move back and impinge on nerves. Another possibility is that—because you became too active too soon, or for some other reason—your back graft never fused completely and so your spine never stabilized as it should have. After some time, it deteriorated to where it was before your operation.

All of these are possible. But today the chances of success of back surgery are about 80 percent, which means the odds are well on your side (no pun intended). They are even heavier in your favor when you know you have a competent, careful surgeon operating in a well-controlled, tightly run community hospital that is dedicated to service and education.

As we said earlier, your physician will recommend surgery only when he is convinced that it is the only resort. And your surgeon will operate on your back only if he feels likewise. Any operation is a serious stress to your body. While modern surgery performs wonders, it is still nothing to take lightly. It taxes the body and brings you temporary discomfort. But when it is the only way to go, it can give you a new way of life that is free of backache, with its permanent and recurrent distress and disability.

# 9. Standing, Sitting, Squatting, Sleeping

The nice thing about having your back in shape is that you can be vertical again. But if you are going to stay vertical without pain you will have to learn how to do things without imposing unnecessary, dangerous and even injurious loads on your troubled back. This will probably mean that you'll have to learn new ways of doing things, that you'll have to break old habits that were bad for your back and replace them with good new habits. It probably means you'll have to revise the way you have been standing most of your life, as well as change the ways you sit, sleep and lift things. You'll need these new habits whether your bad back was treated at home, in a hospital bed or by surgery. Or all three. What you have to learn now is the proper way to do things—with the least stress and strain on your back. These techniques are often called *body mechanics.*

Years ago, one of the nation's leading proponents of body mechanics, Dr. Joel E. Goldthwait of Massachusetts General Hospital, wrote, "In good body mechanics, the weight of the trunk and head rests mostly on the bodies of the vertebrae

and the intervertebral disks. The articular facets normally
act only as stabilizers. . . . No two individuals are built alike
or use their bodies habitually in similar ways. One has only to
stand on a street corner and watch the crowds go by in order
to see how differently people walk. One can realize then that
every spine at every step is receiving a heavy or light jar of the
body weight from the ground."[1]

STANDING. How you stand determines how much strain
you impose on your back when you are vertical. We're talking here about *posture*. Proper posture can save you much
grief from your back, but improper posture can bring on another siege of back trouble.

Good posture is neither a relaxed, slumped-shoulder
stance nor a rigid swayback, shoulders-back stance. In both
of these improper postures the body is out of balance and the
spine either curves forward too much or curves back. Furthermore, these postures impose unusual strains on the muscles and ligaments that support the back.

Chances are that this has happened: as you got older your
stomach relaxed more and sagged. As you developed a "pot,"
your spine at the lower back bent forward slowly but more
sharply, accenting "lordosis." As your tummy starts sagging,
your chest begins to droop and then your shoulders follow.
If you are a woman with large breasts, their weight accen-
tuates this droop. All this puts your back out of balance. To
quote Dr. Goldthwait again, "When the human machine is
out of balance, physiologic function cannot be perfect; muscles and ligaments are in an abnormal state of tension and
strain."

The military-cadet stance of throwing the chest out and
pulling the shoulders back also overemphasizes lordosis. At

[1]Joel E. Goldthwait et al., *Essentials of Body Mechanics in Health and
Disease*, 5th ed. (Philadelphia: J. P. Lippincott, 1952), p. 93.

the same time, it too often ignores the abdominal muscles, which stay flabby. Then, when the "brace"—as this posture is often called—is relaxed, the person often reverts to a slumped posture.

The main principle of healthy posture is a well-aligned spine. This means a spine that doesn't lean to one side and a spine whose curves are normal. It also means that muscles that support the spine are in balance. One of the best ways of achieving good posture is to stand tall. If you stand as tall as you can—without being rigid about it—your low spinal curve will be properly shallow, you'll throw your chest up and out, and you'll pull in your abdominal muscles slightly. And—most important—the whole weight of your body will be straight up-and-down and squarely centered over your feet.

There is a very quick and easy way to check your posture. You should use it every day, even several times a day until you develop the habit of proper posture. Here's how it works:

Stand with your back against a wall. Your heels, your rump, your shoulders and your head should be pressed against the wall. Move one of your hands to feel for any space between the small of your back and the wall. If there is space there, your back is arched too much.

Now shuffle your feet forward and bend your knees so that your back slides a few inches down the wall. Next, tighten your abdominal muscles and your buttock muscles. The idea is to flatten your lower back against the wall. Hold this position and "walk" your feet back so that you will slide up the wall. Then standing straight, walk away from the wall and around the room. Return to the wall and back up to it to see if you have maintained this proper posture.

What this test teaches you is how to rotate your pelvis— tilt it back, really—to achieve a "flat" lower back. In fact, if you think about tilting back your pelvis and do it, you will not only straighten out the curve of your lower spine, but also tighten your abdominal muscles and thus hold your pot belly in.

The next chapter will tell about exercises for strengthening the muscles that will help you to maintain a healthy posture.

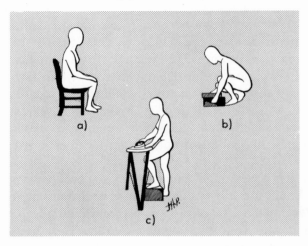

*How to sit, lift, stand. Always keep the small of your back straight when sitting and lifting. When standing, keep one leg raised to keep the tension in the spine and swayback to a minimum.    Fig. 6*

You impose stress on your spine and muscles even when you stand in a proper posture. Fig. 6-C shows a good way to relieve the stress on your back while standing at the ironing board. It would apply equally as well for a man standing at his workbench or counter. The trick is to raise one foot. A footrest thus is a back aid. Lifting one foot serves to flatten the small of the back. (Again! You see it's an important principle.)

The worst way to stand is leaning forward with your hips against the sink, counter, etc. This is liable to force you to hold your shoulders back in order to try to achieve some sort of balance, thereby deepening the curve of your lower back into a swayback configuration. If you use a footrest, however you won't have to lean forward. If there is no footrest around, use the first step of a stool or any other convenient rest. Be careful, though, that your footrest is sturdy and fixed. If you choose a flimsy footrest, or one on wheels or casters, you are liable to add even more troubles to your bad back—an accident.

When you have to bend forward over the bathroom sink or your workbench, bend your knees. Don't lean your elbows on the sink and make a swaying suspension bridge of your back. This will overcurve your spine.

For women only: spikes and other high heels promote swayback as well as unsteadiness. Wear low or moderate heels.

SITTING. You live in a sit-down society. You sit at meals, in your car, watching a movie or television, listening to records, in buses, trains and airplanes, in waiting rooms, at your desk or bench. As a result, chair designers have worked with scientists and engineers trying to fashion an ideal seat, but it still has not been built; there is no universal seat. There will probably never be one because you are built a little differently from anyone else, and he from you. So don't expect to find the ideal seat. Instead, you should learn the basic principles of choosing a good seat and of good sitting practices.

The chair seat must be at a comfortable height from the floor. If it is too high, your back will tend to sway forward. If it is too low, you may have a tendency to slump your shoulders forward and bend your back. The worst kind of seat is an overstuffed or otherwise overly soft sofa, the kind you sink back into. Such luxuriant softness may be kind to your skin, but it is very unkind to your back because it allows it to bend back or flex. Similarly, certain foam rubber sofas and chairs can be too soft and thus nonsupportive.

The best kind of chair for you is a straight hard chair, preferably one that curves forward so as to support your back. A typist's chair should have its back support raised or lowered so that it is right at the small of your back. Technically, according to anthropological engineers, such backrests should not have a lateral curvature deeper than that of a circle 7.3 inches in radius.

Too many people with bad backs sit improperly when they drive. Often they lean forward. This is one of the worst things to do to your back. Your back not only lacks support but is jostled around from side-to-side with the motions of the car over bumps and turns. Instead, your rump should be as far back in the car seat as it can go. One way to promote this is to decrease the distance between your seat and the pedals by moving your seat forward so that your legs aren't stretched straight out ahead of you. Another way you can help your back when you drive (especially if your car seat does not support you in the small of the back) is to buy a back support from an auto supply house. There are several kinds. One is made of a row of wooden slats that are fixed to metal straps that hang over the car seat. Another is a firm cushion that supports the small of your back.

The same two principles apply to sitting as to standing. First, keep your lower back straight. Second, try to relieve the stress on your spine that your legs impose when they are straight.

The best way to sit is with your rump well back in the seat and with your lumbar area supported. Keeping your knees above your hips provides maximum relief because it reduces the physical stress on your spine and on the ligaments and muscles that support it. A contour chair, "Mister Chair."

rocking chair, or other chair that supports the small of your back, enables you to put your feet up and that allows you to lean back, can provide relief and comfort to your back while you are relaxing at reading, listening, viewing or conversing.

Fig. 6-A shows you how to sit in a straight-backed chair when you must lean forward to hear or see better or to work at a desk or typewriter. Again, be sure you keep that lower back straight. Use your hands and arms to help support you by leaning on armrests or on your seat. You can also relieve stress on your back as you lean forward by crossing your legs.

A very bad way to sit is slumped, with your weight resting on the back of your neck and pelvis. This position places severe stress on the small of your back, its muscles, ligaments and vertebrae. Teenagers often sit this way while reading or talking on the telephone. You are justified when you see your youngster slump like this to shout, "Sit up!" The habits he forms now will affect his back for the rest of his life. It's far easier to start a good new habit than to try to break an old and bad habit.

LIFTING. This can get you into more trouble than any other activity involving your back.

As you bend forward from the waist and lift, you are imposing the maximum amount of physical stress on your spine, its ligaments and your back muscles. When you lift improperly, you impose greater pressures on your intervertebral disks *than with any other activity*. This was shown by 1970 studies in Sweden by Dr. Alf Nachemson of the University of Göteborg and Gösta Elfström, a research engineer at the Chalmers University of Technology, also located at Göteborg. They found that lifting the wrong way—with legs straight and back bent at the waist—imposed pressures of more than 500 pounds per square inch on the L3 disk! By comparison, lifting properly imposed a load of only 227 pounds per square inch, or about half the stress. To understand what kind of pressure even proper lifting imposes, you should know that merely standing imposes a stress of 182 pounds per square inch on the L3 disk. (We'll cite more of these Swedish measurements in the next chapter when we discuss exercises that are good and bad for your back.)

With your bad back, you should get in the habit of NOT lifting at all. It is worth the tip to the porter. It is worth the tow truck fee for changing a flat. It is worth the price to your pride of asking your wife or your friend to lift a bag for you.

However, if you absolutely must lift, there is only one way to do it. That is by bending your knees until you are almost in a sitting position—squatting, in fact—and then lifting by standing up. This action uses the large muscles of your thighs instead of the smaller muscles of your back.

Among the greatest boons to proper lifting by women were the miniskirts of the late 1960's and the Hot Pants of 1971. These styles forced women to lift properly if they were to properly preserve their modesty. Not so with the maxis or midis; wearing either of these allowed women to bend forward from the waist and still maintain decorum, even as they exposed their backs to improper stresses.

Lifting properly, from a crouched position, applies not only to lifting heavy weights but to lifting *anything*—whether from floor, ground or car trunk. Making a bed is murderous for your back if you do it bending forward; you'd be better off on your knees. Opening a window is likewise dangerous.

NEVER, but never, lift a heavy object alone. If you must lift a television set or carton or whatever, get someone to help you; then decide in advance who is doing what and moving where and at what pace. Avoid lifting quickly and make no sudden motions while you are carrying a heavy object. Also, keep the object as close to your body as possible. And DON'T lift the heavy object above your head; this action makes your back sway while it places great stress on it—a very dangerous duo.

SLEEPING should afford your back the most rest and comfort. But it will only do so if the sleeping conditions are right. Your spine is most comfortable when it assumes its normal S-curve, as viewed from the side, and its normal straight line, when seen from the front or rear. If sleeping conditions are not right, your spine, its ligaments and your back muscles will be working all night to try to line up your spine into proper position and will certainly *not* be relaxed.

Your weight is not equally spread along your body. Most of the mass of your body is in your hip area, while another large mass is at your shoulders, or slightly below. So, if you sleep on your side on a feather bed or on a very soft mattress, the heaviest parts of you will sink down the farthest; these are, of course, your hips and shoulders. As a result, your spine will be improperly bent in the middle.

If you sleep on your side on the floor or on a board or on a too hard, unconforming mattress, you'll also improperly bend your spine. Your hips and your shoulders act like the towers of a bridge; suspended between them in an unnatural curve is your spine. This is further complicated by the unequal widths of your hips and shoulders.

All night long, as you sleep on a too soft, or too hard surface, your muscles are working to straighten your spine. This tug-of-war goes on as long as you sleep, be it 6, 8 or 10 hours a night. Small wonder that when you wake up, you complain of an achin' back. Small wonder, indeed! Your poor back has been working hard all night and now, without rest, it has to go to work holding you vertical!

There are millions of people in the world who sleep on the floor or on the ground without suffering any back pain. There are also many people—especially in Germany and in other parts of Central Europe—who think themselves lucky to sleep in feather beds and who also do not suffer back trouble. But YOU are not among these people. They have healthy or even super-healthy backs. You do not.

Some people—alas, even some doctors—recommend to their back patients the insertion of a bed board under the mattress. Unfortunately, this has helped the makers of Masonite and other pressed boards, as well as the makers of plywood, far more than it has helped back sufferers. Here's why: pressed board placed under a mattress will simply sag with the mattress. Heavy (3/4-inch) plywood placed under a mattress will not sag, but it can only give the mattress a base to sag to. It will do nothing about preventing the mattress from sagging!

To be helpful, a mattress has to support you and has to yield only enough to allow for the heaviness of your hips and shoulders. This means it has to be properly firm but not rigid, conforming but not soft. If it meets these specifications, your spine will stay straight as you sleep on your side and your muscles will not be struggling all night. Even more importantly, your spine will not get out of line during the night so as to irritate a nerve root and trigger your back into painful and rigid spasm.

A good, firm mattress used to be hard to find in our land of softness and luxury. But not any more. More and more dealers, aware of the need for properly supportive mattresses, are now stocking them. Similarly, buyers for hotels and motels are becoming more aware of the need for good mattresses for their beds. Even so, you can get a sagging hotel bed once in a while. Try out your mattress when you check into a hotel room. If it sags, call the desk and insist on another one or another room. Don't settle for a bed board, which may be offered to you. And don't sleep on that sagging bed.

When you go to buy a mattress that will be most kind to your back, you'll be confronted with an array of kinds, colors and makes. There are really just a few important principles you should know to help you make an intelligent choice from among the numerous possibilities.

One of the first decisions you'll have to make is whether

you want a spring or a foam mattress. Mattresses with steel coil springs inside (inner springs) are the most popular, probably because that's what most people have slept on for most of their lives. Mattresses made of foam have been sold since the 1950's, but are used by fewer and fewer people. The foam is either latex rubber or polyurethane.

Mattresses come in various grades of firmness. Firmness is just one aspect, however. *Conformity* is another. You want a mattress that not only supports your body's weight but that also conforms to your body's contours.

While mattresses can rest on supports or boards, most have box spring foundations. The box spring is simply a box that encloses metal springs. This serves to give more buoyancy and support to your mattress, enabling it to conform. But a worn-out, saggy box spring won't do this.

Finally, you should realize that mattresses and box springs, like cars or other equipment, can wear out. The trouble here

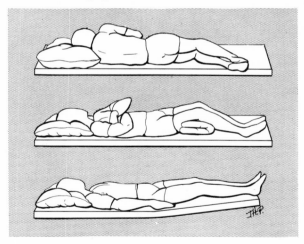

*How to sleep comfortably. Use a firm mattress and assume the semifetal position (top); or on your back with a pillow under your knees (middle); or with your legs raised (bottom).* **Fig. 7**

is that we humans readily adapt to changes in our environment. To feel how you have adapted, go to a bedding store and lie down on a firm new mattress. If you feel a difference, it means you need a mattress. As a rule of thumb (or back), mattresses last about ten years.

Sleeping on your side on a proper mattress, with your legs bent in a sort of semifetal position (à la the curled-up position you assumed in the womb before you were born) can give your back a lot of comfort and rest. But be sure you use a thin pillow under your head to support it. Otherwise it will tilt down and bend your spine improperly. (See top, Fig. 7)

Sleeping on your back either flat or with high pillows under your head induces swayback and can strain your neck, arms and shoulders. If you prefer sleeping on your back, place a pillow or folded blanket under your knees. This relieves the stress on your spine caused by the pull of your legs (middle, Fig. 7). Raising the half of the mattress under your legs has the same effect (bottom, Fig. 7). This has the additional advantage of discouraging you from sleeping on your abdomen.

If you have a hospital-type bed that you can adjust, roll the levers or push the electrical buttons until it is in the gatched, W-like configuration. Then you can sleep on your back in great comfort. Fortunately, these beds are now available to consumers. Unfortunately, they are expensive.

Sleeping on your stomach—whether or not you cuddle with your pillow—is not very good for your back, even on a firm mattress. On a soft mattress, it's murderous. It promotes swayback and strains your back muscles and shoulders. But there is a way to get relief on your stomach: place a thin pillow under your hips. This helps flatten out your back.

It is important that you lie down and get out of bed properly. First, don't do either with any sudden movements. As you go down and get up, your back is vulnerable to injury. Bolting up into the sitting position from lying on your back can be disastrous!

*To lie down:* first sit on the edge of the bed. Then, with your knees and hips still bent in that position, pivot your body on your rump. Put both your hands on the mattress to bear the weight of your trunk as your body pivots and then eases down. When you are down on the mattress you will be on your side in the semifetal position. You can then roll over on to your back, if you like.

*To get up:* Roll over or otherwise get into the semifetal position. Then place your hands on the mattress near your head. Push down with your arms to raise your trunk, as you pivot on your rump with your hips and knees still bent. If you do this smoothly and successfully, you'll find yourself sitting on the edge of your bed. To stand up, bend forward slightly to balance yourself, keeping the small of your back straight; then lift yourself up using mainly your thigh muscles.

Doing things properly is just one aspect of back care, although an important one. You'll also have to learn to strengthen certain muscles. How to do this is the subject of the next chapter.

# 10. The Importance of Exercise

You should always keep in mind the very important fact that your back is erect thanks to a partnership of skeleton and muscles. The skeletal partner is comprised of your vertebrae and disks, the sacrum and pelvis. The muscular partner is made up of ligaments running in front of and behind your spine, and all the muscles and tendons of your trunk, especially those of your back and abdomen.

Just how these partners work together to keep you erect, and to allow you to move around while you are erect, is detailed in Chapter 2. That chapter also explains how in certain conditions—including "slipped" disk and arthritis—these muscles can tighten in painful spasm. The problem here is that a nerve root becomes irritated and the resulting pain triggers the back muscles into tight contraction. This is nature's way of protecting further nerve irritation. But nature here overprotects, the spasm causes more pain, and a bad back attack is the result. You can also suffer an acute back attack by irritating a ligament, muscle or tendon of your back with a sudden movement; this is a sprain. Again, the pain will trigger spasm, which will cause more pain and start the same sort of a cycle.

One of the best ways to avoid further bad back attacks is to get those trunk muscles in shape and keep them in shape. Because the skeletal partner of your back is weakened and having troubles, the muscular partner has to become more dominant. Muscles don't become strong and in good shape by your thinking about them. You have to move them to action; in other words, you have to exercise. And you have to start and continue your personal course of exercise religiously, without fail, without let-up, for the rest of your life. It's small price to pay for many future years of comfort. And regardless of your feelings about exercise now, it is one of the things you *must* do if you are to learn to successfully live with your bad back.

Muscles are wonderful organs of the body. If you don't use them, they wither and shrink, get flabby and lose strength. If you do use them, they stay firm and strong. If you start using unused muscles wisely, they grow and expand, tighten and gain strength. There is some pain associated with restoring flabby muscles, but it is a good kind of pain. It is a sort of ache, really, that lets you know you've done something good for your muscles. And, while it sounds a bit cute, if you do something good for your muscles (exercise them), they'll do something good for your back (keep pain away).

The purpose of exercise is not to make you a Mr. America or a Miss World Olympics. Nor is it to enable you to lift 300 pounds (for heavens sake, don't even try!) or to run the mile faster. The purpose of exercise is twofold:

To educate or train the proper muscles so that you can maintain the proper posture at all times, especially at the small of your back;
To give appropriate muscles the strength they need to give you good posture and to support your troublesome

spine in various positions and activities, without strain and stress.

When we spoke about bones and muscles a few paragraphs above, we only mentioned nerves in passing. Actually, they are very important, especially in exercising. Nerves have to be involved in an automatic, reflex way if you are to keep the proper posture at all times. You can't consciously be thinking about posture all the time. Good posture has to become an automatic behavior that occurs as a reflex, far below the level of your consciousness. In other words, you have to eventually keep the small of your back properly flat, even without thinking about it. This means you'll have to think about it at first, just as when you first do the back-to-wall test described in the previous chapter. But as you keep repeating it, it'll soon develop into a habit. And that's what you should strive for. Keep assuming the proper position and it will soon feel comfortable, while the old crouch or swayback will feel uncomfortable, or at least not quite right. Similarly, the exercises you do to help your back will also teach your nerves and your muscles how to assume the correct position for your back and, if the back is not in the proper configuration, how to move to assume it.

The purpose of exercise is not just to move parts of your body and fan the air. Which exercises you do, how you do them and the number of times you repeat them are what count. Done properly, exercises will strengthen the right muscles in the right ways. Exercises will also educate nerves to automatically tell the muscles to move in the right ways whenever that is necessary. The result should then be less pressure on your troublesome disk or vertebral joint.

Don't jump into exercise like a frog into water, especially if you are out of shape and haven't done any exercise or taken part in athletics in ages. Even if you are in shape, you should take it easy with these special back exercises, because you

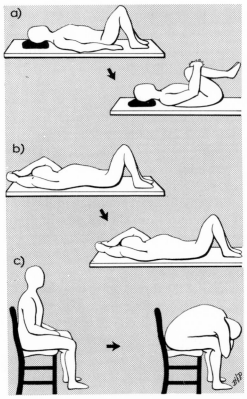

*Back exercises. a.) On your back, with a pillow under your head and arms at your side, raise your knees slowly to your chest. Bring your hands up to clasp your knees. Hold for the count of 10. Do three times. Relax. Repeat. b.) On your back with your knees raised and bent, and your hands above your head. Relax. Then tighten the muscles of your stomach and buttocks at the same time—so as to flatten your back against the floor or mat. Hold for the count of 10. Relax and repeat. c.) Sit on a hard chair with your arms folded loosely in your lap. Let your torso drop forward until your head is between your knees. Then slowly pull your body up erect to a sitting position. Tighten your abdominal muscles as you do so. Relax. Repeat.* **Fig. 8**

probably will be using some muscles in new ways. The result of being too enthusiastic can be muscle sprain. On the other hand, you should approach your exercises with some enthusiasm so that you put into them all the necessary energy and precision.

At the beginning it is better for you to do each exercise, say, five times a day for half a minute each time, than to do it five times in a solid 2½ minutes. The point is to avoid fatigue. You have to get your muscles in condition by stages, starting in short mild exercise periods and gradually building up to longer and more intense exercise periods and then even to athletic activities that supplement the exercises.

The kinds of exercises you should do will probably be explained to you in detail by your doctor. Follow his instructions to the letter, since he'll know best which exercises your bad back specifically needs.

In Fig. 8 you have the three back exercises most commonly prescribed by doctors for their back patients. Each of these exercises is designed to help you to tone up your trunk muscles, thereby relieving the stress on your lower back. Again, that means that you have to learn to tilt your pelvis back and hold it there, thereby counteracting swayback, or lordosis. To tilt your pelvis back you have to use a combination of muscles in your lower abdomen and hips.

All these exercises fall under the category of *isotonic*, which means they are exercises of motion against resistance. The resistance here is twofold: gravity and opposing muscles.

There is another category of exercises, called *isometric exercise*, which involves the pitting of one muscle against another, or against a solid object like a wall, without any motion being produced. Charles Atlas made this popular in the 1930's as Dynamic Tension, a way 97-pound weaklings could build themselves up to fight beach bullies. Then in the 1960's it was revived and modified and made popular again as *isometrics*. The technique involves, for instance, contracting your biceps and triceps of your upper arm at the same time for about six seconds, or trying to push the wall down.

In general, motion exercises (isotonic) are better for your back than static (isometric) exercises because they involve joint motion. Your joints—and that includes spinal joints—are meant to move by sliding and rotating and they are kept healthier by such actions. This is less true in the case of arthritis, however, where bone spurs can cause pain. But even in arthritis, lack of joint movement can accelerate stiffness.

There is one important exception here about isotonics versus isometrics: your abdominal muscles. Merely contracting these as hard as you can and keeping this contraction for about half a minute does wonders toward tightening and strengthening them. This can only help your back as a result. You should tighten your stomach regularly every day. If you drive to work or to shopping, make a habit of doing this tightening exercise every time you stop for a red light. Or do it on the train. Suck in your belly as tight as you can and tighten those muscles and hold it until the light turns green. Hold it . . . hold it. . . .

It's important enough to repeat: get into your exercise routine gradually. Start by trying out each exercise slowly and carefully. Do your horizontal exercises on a carpeted floor and place a thin pillow or folded blanket under your head if you find it more comfortable. You can even do some exercises in bed. Start slowly to warm up your muscles. You can speed up and intensify later. Breathe deeply and synchronize your breathing to the exercise motions. Thus, if you are curling your knees up into your belly and squeezing your chest, exhale; and when you let your legs down and can expand your chest, inhale.

In addition to those exercises shown in Fig. 8, there are two others that can be of benefit to you. One is to lie on your back with your legs drawn up so that your knees are bent in the air. Move your right leg—still bent—toward your chest as you, in opposition, straighten out your left leg. Then return to the starting position and raise the left leg as you straighten the right.

The other exercise involves standing behind a chair or facing a table or desk. While holding on to the table, chair, or desk, lower yourself into the squatting position with your lower back bent only slightly. Then, while maintaining that configuration of your back, lift yourself up again to a standing position, using your thigh muscles to do so.

As your muscles become firm and gain strength, you'll notice that the exercises become easier and less painful, both while you're doing them and afterward. You may very well feel so good that you want to do more active and more strenuous exercises, or even engage in your favorite sport. You should always check first with your doctor before you change your exercise program. He will probably advise you to next start a program of mild calisthenics as the second step.

In calisthenics, you have to be very careful to warm up properly, to start slowly and to take it easy at first. Your doctor and you also have to very carefully select the proper calisthenics. They are not innocuous; some can be harmful, in fact. Among the most harmful and the ones you should avoid are those that flex the back—make you bend forward, in other words. If you look at Tables 1 and 2, you can get some idea of how much pressure these kinds of exercises place on your disks.

We should explain these charts before we go on. As we explained in the previous chapter, they are derived from experiments performed in Sweden by a physician and engineer. The data were selected from among the many measurements this Swedish pair performed on healthy human volunteers—healthy, specifically, in terms of their backs. The measurements were made during various physical activities by means of tiny electronic devices implanted by needle into each vol-

TABLE 1

PRESSURES INSIDE THE HEALTHY L3 INTERVERTE-
BRAL DISK OF A WOMAN WITH NO BACK TROUBLE

AGE: 24 Years        HEIGHT: 5 ft. 6 in.
WEIGHT: 126 lb.

| *ACTIVITY* | *PRESSURE* |
|---|---|
| Traction, supine | 40 lb./sq. in. |
| Prone | 57 |
| Supine | 57 |
| Traction, standing | 71 |
| Crook-lying relaxed | 85 |
| Passive back hyperextension | 85 |
| Upright standing | 100 |
| Sitting, no support | 120 |
| Walking | 120 |
| Upright standing, 22 lb. in each hand | 135 |
| Bilateral straight leg raising | 149 |
| Jumping | 150 |
| Laughing | 164 |
| Straining | 164 |
| Coughing | 174 |
| Contraction of abdominal muscle against resistance | 177 |
| Twisting, 22 lb. in each hand | 185 |
| Bending sideways, 22 lb. in each hand | 192 |
| Lifting of 44 lb. with bending of knees | 206 |
| Bending forward 30° | 214 |
| Active back hyperextension | 228 |
| Sit-up with knees bent | 256 |
| Sit-up with knees extended | 256 |
| Bending forward 30°, 22 lb. in each hand | 281 |
| Sitting, leaning forward, 22 lb. in each hand | 300 |
| Lifting of 44 lb. with bending of back | 384 |

[Adapted from Table **IV**, *Intravital Dynamic Pressure Measurements in Lumbar Disks,* by Alf Nachemson, M.D., and Gosta Elfström, M.Sc.Eng. Almquist & Wiksell, Stockholm, 1970. Published as Supplement No. 1 to *Scandinavian Journal of Rehabilitation Medicine.*]

## TABLE 2

### CHANGE IN LOAD ON L3 DISK, BY PERCENTAGES
### (STANDING IS 100%)

| ACTIVITIES | 0 | 100 | 200 | 300 | 400 |
|---|---|---|---|---|---|
| Standing | | | | | |
| Lying | | | | | |
| Walking | | | | | |
| Twisting | | | | | |
| Bending to the Side | | | | | |
| Coughing | | | | | |
| Jumping | | | | | |
| Straining | | | | | |
| Laughing | | | | | |
| Lifting Correctly | | | | | |
| Forward Bending, 44 lb. in Hands | | | | | |
| Lifting Incorrectly | | | | | |
| *EXERCISES* | | | | | |
| Isometric Contraction of Abdominal Muscles | | | | | |
| Lifting Both Legs | | | | | |
| Active Back Hyperextended | | | | | |
| Sit-up, Knees Extended | | | | | |
| Sit-up, Knees Bent | | | | | |

[Adapted from Figure 20, *Intravital Dynamic Pressure Measurements in Lumbar Disks,* by Alf Nachemson, M.D., and Gosta Elfström, M.Sc.Eng. Almquist & Wiksell, Stockholm, 1970. Published as Supplement No. 1 to *Scandinavian Journal of Rehabilitation Medicine.*]

unteer's L3 disk. These devices (*transducers,* in electronic jargon) detected and measured pressures in the interior of the disk and broadcast their readings to a specially built and very sensitive radio.

To give you some idea of the tremendous pressures imposed on your own lumbar disks during these various activities, we chose the data in Table 1 from tests on a slim, young woman. (We also converted from metric measures to pounds and inches.)

Looking at Table 1, you can see that sit-ups impose some

of the highest disk pressures recorded by the Swedish researchers: 256 pounds per square inch (lb./sq. in.)! To give you reference points, lying down imposed only 57 lb./sq. in., and standing 100. To give you a mechanical comparison, the cylinder compression pressure inside the engine of an English sports car (an MG-B) is 160 lb./sq. in. More exactly, the pressure in a disk when you perform a sit-up is the same crushing pressure that a steel submarine has to withstand at a depth of 570 feet below the surface of the ocean!

If you study Table 1 closely, you can get a good understanding of the kinds of calisthenics and other exercises you need to stay away from.

For a faster comparison, look at Table 2. It is a bar graph that shows percentages of pressure increases with various activities.

To make things easier, here is a list of some *calisthenics to avoid*:

| | |
|---|---|
| toe-touches | straight leg raises (both together) |
| hip twists | toes over head |
| sit-ups | upside-down bicycle |

Don't misunderstand. There are some calisthenics that are very good for your back, that you should do every day when you are in shape. One is the *push-up*. This exercise is excellent for building up and keeping in tone the muscles of the front of your trunk, especially those of the abdomen and upper chest. You should do 30. The *knee bend* is good for strengthening thighs; just be careful not to sink all the way down as this can endanger your hamstring muscles by overstretching them. Also, be sure that when you do this exercise that your back is flat.

*Side straddle hop* is a good general exercise. Just be sure you land each time on your toes so that you don't give your back too sharp a jolt with each hop. Do 20.

The *chin-up* is a good exercise because it helps tighten abdominal muscles as it tightens those of the upper trunk. Do 10.

The chin-up also provides traction to relieve pressure on your spine; as you hang by your hands, the weight of your pelvis and legs pulls on your spine. In fact, the Swedish measurements showed that such vertical traction reduces to a minimum the pressure inside a disk. Some doctors recommend hanging by the hands or arms even to people who do not have the strength to pull their chins up to the bar. Most important here is that the feet clear the floor. If the bar or trapeze swings a bit, you will find it easier to hang on since that keeps changing the muscle tensions of the arms.

According to an article in *Medical Times* of March, 1970, by Dr. Edward L. McNeil of New York, "The swing is not practical for the acute case. Its most useful application is perhaps in the convalescent stage and as a prophylactic measure in patients who are liable to frequent recurrences. . . ." In his view, "The slight overswing of the feet in relationship to the spine is considered to rhythmically and alternately stretch the spinal flexors and extensors. The weight of the legs and pelvis represents an excellent traction force aided by gravity."

There are sports, games and athletic activities that can help your back, but there are others that can harm it. The sports to avoid are those in which there is rough physical contact, where there is dangerous physical stress to your back, where there is twisting and where there is the danger of sudden impact. That means that the sports you should *stay away from* include:

|                   |                          |
| ----------------- | ------------------------ |
| basketball        | sledding and tobogganing |
| boat rowing       | snowmobiling             |
| bowling           | soccer                   |
| diving            | trampoline               |
| football          | tennis                   |
| handball          | volleyball               |
| high-jumping      | weight lifting           |
| pole vaulting     |                          |

Another group of sports is in a gray area of sometimes

good, sometimes bad. If you are skilled at the game and do it with proper form and coordination, it is okay. But if you are unskilled and uncoordinated, you can do your back a great deal of harm. Included in this category are:

baseball
golf
horseback riding
ice skating (not hockey)
jogging and running (if you can
    control your lordosis)

karate
jujitsu
skiing (water and snow)
wrestling

*Swimming* is at the top of the list of sports that you can and should take part in. In the first place, the water buoys you and you are horizontal, both of which means that there is a minimum of pressure on your disks or joints to keep your back erect. Also, swimming involves just about all the muscles you want to get involved. Furthermore, you don't have to rely on an opponent or teammate; you can go swimming on your own on a regular basis. But that does not mean you can perform high diving or any other kind from a board. This is absolutely out because of the jerk your spine receives when you hit the water.

Swimming does, however, include *skin diving*—that is underwater swimming with the aid of face mask, snorkel and fins. *Scuba diving*, per se, with the use of an air tank and regulator is all right, only if you don't try to walk around with the tank belted to your back. In the water the tank is at neutral buoyancy, so there is no stress on your back; but on land that's a lot of weight for your back to hold up, which means it may worsen your lordosis.

*Hiking* is a very good activity for your back. Just don't strap on a big field pack or scale any steep heights. And be careful of iced and slippery pavements. *Bicycling* is also good —but keep your back straight!

If you have a question about any specific sport or exercise, ask your doctor. But you probably have a proper feeling for what is good and what is bad for your back by what we've said so far. We want to be sure that this does not frighten you or keep you from getting in shape and exercising regularly, or from regularly taking part in some suitable sport. Men and women who engage in sports have better muscle tone—specifically of the trunk muscles. What's more, they feel better; they are limber and the very physical activity lends a psychological boost by reducing nervous tension. So exercisers are happier in general.

All of these are reasons you should exercise—and regularly.

In many ways and for many back sufferers, their troubles result from an overly comfortable way of life that has led to deterioration of their muscles and, as a result, of the way they stand, sit, lift, walk and otherwise move. Most boys are physically active while they are in school and perhaps for a few years after—particularly if they are in the military service. Then, as men, their activity falls off to one picnic baseball game or a round or two of golf in the summer.

The situation is usually even softer and less strenuous for the female in our society. If you are a woman, the chances are that you were never physically active: you could never even do one push-up, for instance.

We could probably stem the tide of bad backs in our society if we got our youngsters physically fit, and ingrained in them an understanding of the need for constantly staying fit, as well as of the joys and benefits of exercise and sports. We should teach our youngsters proper posture, as well as the proper way to sit and lift and sleep. But before that, we have to teach the teachers how these are properly done. Too many teachers don't know—unless they have suffered a bad back and have had to learn for themselves. We also need to change some of our social values. We need to promote such beneficial activities as ballet, which teaches proper posture and grace; while downgrading such glorious but injurious and dangerous sports as boxing and football. At the same time, we have to emphasize participation in sports and deemphasize the passive pastime of the flabby sports fan who sits in front of a television set all weekend and on holidays.

Also, we should stop mechanizing sports. There is little exercise in golf today, as players ride from shot to shot sitting in golf carts, instead of walking the links as the game was meant to be played. Even skiing has lost its vigor, thanks to chair lifts. With rope tows, skiers got some exercise; with the old way of climbing up the grade, they got even more.

Finally, after you've exercised or played your game, you may feel like a warm bath, a hot shower, a steam bath or even a sauna. Any of these is good. Heat helps *you* to relax and does wonders to make your muscles relax. So does a good massage. Just two bits of advice here: it is traditional in Turkish baths to douse yourself with cold water once the heat becomes unbearable. Don't do it. The shock of that water can trigger a reflex jerking of your back that could cause great pressures and problems. For the same reason, don't turn on the cold water as a finish to your hot shower. Leave it hot and walk away from the shower with relaxed muscles. Also, most steam and sauna baths provide only wooden slats to sit on, with no back supports. Watch yourself and be sure you sit with your back flat; or, better yet, lie down—but be careful not to fall asleep in that suffocating heat.

Above all, keep those back and abdominal muscles in shape. The time you spend each day exercising is a small investment toward preventing time lost from work and play with another back attack. Besides, you'll look and feel better.

# 11. Emotions and Your Back

Your bad back is a very emotional condition: it can deeply affect your emotions and your emotions can deeply affect it.

Probably the overwhelming emotion provoked by the sharp pain and by the serious disability that comes with a back attack is fear. Having once gone through a back attack, some people turn into "back cripples."

Lying there during an attack, every movement of your trunk filled with pain, is enough to scare anyone. So no bad back sufferer need ever be ashamed of that fear he or she has experienced. You begin to wonder at such times if you'll ever be vertical again, if you'll ever be able to walk again, if you'll ever be able to do any of the things you like doing as an active person.

Lying there, you wonder who is taking care of your family; you worry about all the small details you always attend to every day that you've never told anyone else about. You remember the stories told by your friends who have had back trouble and you imagine some of these same things happening to you. You may even find yourself starting to feel some of the same pains or numbness they described to you about their situation.

As you get better, you may have a new worry. "All right," you say, "I'm recovering pretty well from this one. Now, when is the next attack going to hit? Will I forever live under this Sword of Damocles that is pointed at my lower back?"

So, fearful of pain and disability striking again, many back patients become depressed and moody. Some figure, "The heck with it; I won't do anything. That way I won't provoke it." Such back cripples spend most of their time sitting (improperly), even afraid to take walks for fear of aggravating yet another attack.

Even your doctor can't tell you whether you'll have another back attack, although the chances are that once you've had one bad back incident, you'll have others. But only by exercising, practicing the proper postural habits and body mechanics as described in the previous chapters, and by taking care of yourself, generally can you keep holding off that next attack. Doing nothing and, even worse, falling back into sloppy posture and improper sitting, sleeping and lifting practices can shorten the time between attacks.

People who have had surgery on their back and then continue to have pain and/or numbness can also become crippled by their emotions. Too many of them hadn't believed their surgeons who warned them before their operation that they would not be totally free of pain immediately afterward. The public still tends to look upon surgery as miraculous. It may be wonderful, but it is not magical. Frequently there are remnants of back pain in the weeks and even months following surgery (as we explained in Chapter 8). It takes time for nerve roots to get back to normal after years of pressure and torture. Also, during your operation microscopic nerve fibers may have become entrapped in scar tissue. Scar tissue keeps contracting, which means it pulls on the nerves, producing pain. With all these unseen, but very

much felt biological processes going on, you should expect
your pain and/or numbness to completely disappear only
after about 18 months. However, you can resume most of
your activities long before then.

It's easy to understand how pain can make you afraid that
the operation went wrong; however, if you keep these facts
in mind, your fear should lessen, and your activities increase.

The next time you feel frightened about your back, do
something, don't just lie there. And the something you do
should be a posture check or a helpful exercise.

You are also going to have to face the fact, and face it
squarely, that your back is always going to ache you sometime. People with bad backs go through periods when their
backs give them no trouble, and yet at other times they could
wish them on their worst enemy, as the saying goes. Curse
and bear it, if that helps. You will also find that a strong mo-
tivation to do something can overcome your pain. Many people with bad backs who shouldn't be playing tennis, for instance, do so and feel wonderful while they are on the courts.
Yet when they stop, their backs hurt again. These players
realize that pain is the price they have to pay for playing, yet
they are willing to pay that price.

Too many people with bad backs are so fearful that they
don't engage in sex with their mates. To our minds, this is
carrying things much too far. We know of no reported case
of a back going into acute spasm during coitus.

You're going to have to get over the shock that comes
with the realization that you are not perfect. That blunt statement itself may come as a shock. Still, physicians recognize
that just about everyone (themselves included) thinks of himself as infallible and invulnerable. Then, when he is struck
down with a bad back, his ego is bruised. As he realizes the
chronic nature of his condition, he is also chagrined to realize
that he will never be perfect again. This can make many peo-

ple fearful and apprehensive. Just recognize that *no one* is perfect. Even great people have feet of clay—and backaches. Only deity, never humanity, can be flawless!

The opposite of what we have been saying is also true. Emotions influence your back and its pain. Again, take sex. As we said earlier in this book, there are patients who have difficulty with their partners, or with their own arousal, who blame their backs. "Not tonight, dear, my back is killing me" is a familiar put-off in such circumstances. It is also a psychological put-off to keep you from painful social occasions. The point is that the back can be the whipping post of your emotions. The pain is just as real when it is caused by psychosomatic reasons as when it is caused by arthritis, slipped disk or pulled muscle. That's one reason you should never diagnose yourself, and it's the reason that good doctors never make spot diagnoses, but instead talk to and carefully examine their patients.

Your back is your "medical thing," the part of your body that at times is most responsive to your moods and emotional feelings. Everybody has a "medical thing." Some have ulcers. You have a painful back. Having problems at work? Nervous over a big business deal? Angry at your wife? Your back aches!

This may not be true of you, but there are people who use their backache to almost totally withdraw from other people. If they are unhappy with their mate or impotent or frigid, backache is the mechanism. If they are very depressed and want to get away from everyone, backache from unknown cause is an excuse for being sent to another world, that of the hospital.

Again, this probably doesn't apply to you, but there are neurotics who use their backs to manipulate other people. These are the patients who make the rounds and go from one doctor to another, always starting their story at the beginning and seldom letting on at first that they have been to other doctors before. These people are often looking for a doctor who can serve as a father-figure, someone who can control them. But they are uncontrollable.

You can see how we are leading up to the idea that doctors who specialize in orthopedics may occasionally refer their patients to colleagues who specialize in the treatment of emotional disorders. If your doctor senses that you have an emotional problem tied up with your back, he may very well suggest that you see a psychiatrist or a psychiatric social worker to identify and treat the problem. Many are the jokes about psychiatrists, for widespread is the fear of them. To many people they are still unknown and mysterious. Yet these specialists of emotional disabilities are as well-equipped to take care of patients as are specialists of physical disabilities.

There should be no shame at all associated with a doctor's referring his patient to a psychiatrist. Rather, there should be relief at the prospect that help may be on the way, that at long last the problem may be pinpointed and worked on, and hopefully solved by one means or another, be it tranquilizers or psychotherapy.

All the same, psychiatry won't cure a backache, so don't think that a few sessions with a psychiatrist will make the pain go away. It will, instead, identify the kinds of emotional problems linked with the pain and may ultimately result in permanent relief.

Some people even use their back as a way of getting money. When someone consciously imitates a bad back condition and sets about trying to collect by insurance or legal suit, this is a type of malingering. Sometimes this is done as a way of capitalizing on an auto accident case. None of this need apply to you, but you ought to know there are people like this who muddy the legal waters for honest back sufferers. Such persons are a major reason that insurance rates keep rising beyond those caused by inflation alone. As the doctor's magazine, *Medical World News,* pointed out (May 7, 1971), "Some insurers are starting to treat back pain claims in their own way—with money. They are offering outright cash settlements, leaving the claimant, should he take the lump sum, free to shop around for therapy" or not.

Not many doctors would agree with Los Angeles psychiatrist Dr. Charles Wahl, who contends that 90 percent of backaches are basically due to deep-seated emotional problems that cause trouble-triggering tightening of muscles in the spinal region. Still, it is a fact that nervous tensions cause tightness of muscles. So this must be one of the causes of backache.

Muscle relaxants and tranquilizers serve to take the tightness out of these muscles. But so does proper exercise. Again, exercise has not only a good physical effect on your body but a sound and exhilarating effect on your nerves, releasing as it does nervous tension that is manifested as tight muscles. Thus relaxation is the result of exercise .

This means that a few push-ups or laps of the pool can often be as helpful as a few pills. Even more so, since such exercise also keeps your muscles in shape. Furthermore, you are psychologically uplifted by your accomplishment.

As we said at the beginning of this chapter, your back affects your emotions and your emotions affect your back. It's all part of the same totality that is your bad back. Recognizing the tug of war between spine and mind is a big step toward learning to successfully live with your bad back.

# 12. Living with Yourself

Your bad back will not kill you, but if it goes into another attack, the pain may get so bad that you may think of death. But it will only be a fleeting wish for the unthinkable. Living, even with that back, is far more preferable. The hellishness of it is that, unlike the pain that comes with infection, in the midst of back pain you are quite alert and quite conscious, and therefore aware of every flame of pain that licks at your back and perhaps also your legs.

Fear of another attack, as we explained in the previous chapter, can so emotionally affect some back sufferers that they become back cripples who withdraw into their emotional cocoons, attempting nothing physical. Other patients so resent the idea of their backs "taking control" over them, that they just do anything they please as though to taunt and challenge their backs to just dare go into another spasm.

Both of these attitudes are extremes and actually are purely psychological ways for coping with the situation of a bad back. One way is to succumb to, the other to deny the existence of, back trouble. Each is as irrational as the other. And each can only lead to more extensive problems than any reasonable, rational approach.

The point is that the sooner you face your back problem squarely and honestly, the sooner you will be on the road to living with it successfully. And you have to do just that: live with it. Your back trouble will simply not disappear. You cannot divorce yourself from it. You may as well recognize that fact and save yourself a lot of suffering, rather than reaching that conclusion only after several bad back bouts. Adjust, prepare and ride out your problem.

As we said, your back condition is not dangerous to life. But it may last your life. Even if you have had surgery, there will be times when it will ache, when it will drag you down, when it will keep you from doing things. Whether or not you really want to do these things is something you'll have to have second thoughts about since, as we explained in the last chapter, there is interplay between your emotions and your back.

If you want to expect the best performance from your back in the years ahead, you are going to have to take the little extra trouble required to take care of it. This means (as we have detailed in previous chapters) that you are going to have to

—exercise regularly
—relax in hot tub or shower regularly
—practice proper posture by standing high and sitting with your back properly supported
—sleep on a firm mattress, curled on your side or lying on your back with a pillow under your legs
—avoid lifting; if you must, do so from a crouched position, using your leg muscles
—keep your weight down to normal
—recognize that your back is your emotional weathervane.

If you are pregnant, you have special circumstances and require more rest for your back.

You are going to have to learn to live with the rest of yourself, too.

You are going to have to resign yourself to the realization that some set of circumstances of mind and body will provoke another bad back attack at some time in the future. Your back may go into a lovely, livable period of quiet. It happened to Ted. He just woke up one day and felt no pain. During such a painfree state you may (as he did) easily delude yourself into thinking that nothing is wrong with your back anymore. These can be comfortable, active months (or even years), free as they are of pain and anguish and disability. But try to keep in the back of your mind the realization that it will all go wrong again some time in the future. We don't say this to frighten you or to take the bloom off this nice pain-free era. We only want you to be realistic about yourself and about your back, so that when it comes, you won't be too surprised or too shaken.

In a way, you have to assume an attitude similar to that of successful diabetics: that you are going to live with your condition and enjoy life by adjusting your living, your habits and your attitudes to your condition. You only cheat yourself if you try to break the rules your doctor has set for your back care.

You have to also realize that in many ways your back attacks are the result of stressful living; and so one way to stave off that next attack is to reduce the nervous stress in your life. You should start enjoying life and stop punishing yourself with meeting people and doing things you don't really like to do, with taking on jobs and assignments that you don't really enjoy. You have to start proportioning your days and weeks to leave enough time for pleasurable pursuits of life. You also need time for exercise and for relaxation. If you deny yourself these, you shortchange your back.

You also have to learn to express yourself. If you are unhappy, say so. If someone irritates you, tell him or her so. That includes your mate. It helps to blow your top once in a while. That's what sensitivity training is all about: to help people learn that it is all right to express their feelings about other people and to hear the opinions of others about themselves.

You also have to learn to worry only about the things you can influence. You would be wise to adopt the code of Alcoholics Anonymous. It has a universal application:

> God grant me the serenity to accept those things
>   I cannot change,
> The courage to change those things I can,
> And the wisdom to know the difference.

Traveling can present special problems and anxieties for back sufferers. There is always the possibility that your back might go into spasm on a trip when you are far from home.

To put your mind at ease, take along the right supplies. If you have a corset or other back appliance, take it. Even if you haven't used it in years, pack it in your bag. You never know when you might need it. Also ask your doctor for the name of a colleague in the towns you visit; there is nothing as reassuring as knowing whom to call in an emergency away from home.

You should also pack any muscle relaxant medicines your doctor has prescribed, although be sure not to take them if you are driving, since they can make you drowsy and you don't want to fall asleep at the wheel.

Also, if you drive, be sure you follow the advice given in Chapter 9 about a back support and moving the seat forward. Also, follow the advice there about hotel beds.

One of the most solid bits of advice we can give train and plane travelers is: hire a red cap, skycap, porter or bellhop to take your luggage. Lifting those bags can impose lots of unnecessary physical stress on your lumbar back. No matter how many transfers you make from taxi to plane or train or bus to hotel, the small charge or tips you'll pay will be worth the savings in stress on your back.

There is nothing like a hot bath at the end of a day of

travel. It does wonders to relax your muscles as well as to rest your mind. And if you have a choice of locations for your vacation, choose a warm climate with a spot near the sea or with a pool. There is nothing like floating or swimming in warm water to ease that back of yours. The antithesis is snowmobiling and the shock and cold it subjects backs to.

Likewise shoveling snow. Get yourself a power snowblower or hire a young neighbor to shovel for you. Bending over and then lifting the snow is absolutely murder for your back. It imposes on it the maximum amount of physical stress. So don't shovel snow. It's that simple.

When you are in these periods of grace when your back feels comfortable, you will probably try to do things you shouldn't be doing. The best advice is: resist the temptation. If you do fall to the temptation, however, lie down afterward and let your back recover. Better yet, take a hot bath and let your entire back relax. This is a good form of preventive medicine you can practice on your own. Similarly, whenever your back starts to ache, lie down, take a hot bath and go lie down again. You may even take a day or two off from work to rest your back. Sure you'll get impatient, but remember the day or two you "waste" this way can save weeks and months of disability. A day of prevention, in other words, is worth a month of treatment.

You should practice relaxation not only on vacation but at various times during your day. Working at your job or at home chores can tighten up your back muscles as you concentrate on your tasks. Stop, get up and walk around; or get down and do some exercises; or sit down and have a cup of coffee. Do this at least in midmorning and at midafternoon. Just five minutes at a time away from work can go a long way toward breaking up the tightness in your back. You see, all your back needs is a break, a chance to relax once in a while.

Developing a sense of humor is another way to relieve the stresses on your back. We realize that these are serious and tense times we live in. But think a minute and you will realize that throughout history man has lived under stress and danger. Lord Houghton wrote, "The sense of humor is the just balance of all the faculties of man, the best security against the pride of knowledge and the conceits of the imagination, the strongest inducement to submit with a wise and pious patience to the vicissitudes of human existence."

You should not at all feel bad about striving for happiness. What else are we on earth for? As Robert Louis Stevenson wrote, "There is no duty we underrate so much as the duty of being happy." The great Cicero said, "To be content with our own is the greatest and most certain wealth of all."

Be happy, and your back will be happy. Take care of your back, and it will hold you erect as long as you live. Know yourself, and you will know your back. Be good to yourself, and your back will be good to you.

# Index

147